THE
DANIEL PRAYER

PRAYER THAT MOVES HEAVEN AND CHANGES NATIONS

STUDY GUIDE + STREAMING VIDEO

SIX SESSIONS

ANNE GRAHAM LOTZ

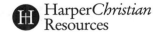
HarperChristian Resources

THE
DANIEL
PRAYER

STUDY GUIDE + STREAMING VIDEO

Books by Anne Graham Lotz

Jesus Followers

Jesus In Me

The Daniel Prayer: Prayer That Moves Heaven and Changes Nations

Wounded by God's People: Discovering How God's Love Heals Our Hearts

Expecting to See Jesus: A Wake-Up Call for God's People

The Magnificent Obsession: Embracing the God-Filled Life

God's Story

Just Give Me Jesus

Pursuing More of Jesus

Why? Trusting God When You Don't Understand

Heaven: My Father's House (revised)

The Vision of His Glory: Finding Hope in the Revelation of Jesus Christ

Video Bible Studies by Anne Graham Lotz

Jesus Followers (Study Guide + Streaming Video and DVD)

Jesus In Me (Study Guide + Streaming Video and DVD)

The Daniel Prayer (Study Guide + Streaming Video and DVD)

Expecting to See Jesus (Study Guide and DVD)

The Magnificent Obsession (Study Guide and DVD)

God's Story (Study Guide and DVD)

Pursuing More of Jesus (Study Guide and DVD)

Heaven (Curriculum DVD and Children's DVD)

The Vision of His Glory (Study Guide and DVD)

For more resources by Anne Graham Lotz visit
www.AnneGrahamLotz.org

CONTENTS

ABOUT ANNE GRAHAM LOTZ

Called "the best preacher in the family" by her father, Billy Graham, Anne Graham Lotz speaks around the globe with the wisdom and authority of years spent studying God's Word.

The *New York Times* named Anne one of the five most influential evangelists of her generation. She's been profiled on *60 Minutes* and has appeared on TV programs such as *Larry King Live, The Today Show,* and *Hannity Live.* Her *Just Give Me Jesus* revivals have been held in more than thirty cities in twelve different countries, to hundreds of thousands of attendees.

Whether a delegate to Davos' Economic Forum, a commentator to the *Washington Post,* or a groundbreaking speaker on platforms throughout the world, Anne's aim is clear—to bring revival to the hearts of God's people. And her message is consistent—calling people into a personal relationship with God through His Word and through prayer.

In May 2016, Anne was named the Chairperson of the National Day of Prayer Task Force, a position held by only two other women, Shirley Dobson and Vonette Bright, since its inception in 1952.

Anne is a bestselling and award-winning author. Her most recent releases are *Jesus Followers, The Light of His Presence, Jesus in Me, The Daniel Prayer, Wounded by God's People, Fixing My Eyes on Jesus, Expecting to See Jesus,* and her first children's book, *Heaven: God's Promise for Me.*

Anne and her late husband, Danny Lotz, have three grown children and three grandchildren. She is the founder and president of AnGeL Ministries, an independent, non-profit organization based in Raleigh, North Carolina, that is committed to giving out messages of biblical exposition so God's Word is personal and relevant to ordinary people.

The ministry's name is derived from the initials of Anne Graham Lotz (AGL) and is especially fitting, as angels are messengers of God who go wherever He sends, speak to whomever He directs, and faithfully deliver His Word. AnGeL Ministries serves as the umbrella organization for the diverse ministry of Anne Graham Lotz—including her many books, DVDs, CDs, speaking engagements, and special events.

To learn more about Anne and AnGeL Ministries, visit

www.annegrahamlotz.org

PREFACE

Do you ever long for a more effective prayer life? Have you ever become so discouraged that you wanted to give up even trying? I have!

I'm reminded of an old CD player I once had. Its carousel would take five CDs at a time. One day when I loaded it, it refused to play the CDs. When I pushed the button for it to eject them, nothing happened. So I banged and pried on the little door, but to no avail. I took it to the shop, and the technician said he would have it fixed in three days. When I went back to get it, the man said, "Mrs. Lotz, I'm sorry. I couldn't get it to work. I did break it open to get your CDs out, but the player won't work." So I threw it away.

When something doesn't fulfill its purpose, it's useless. Is that how you have come to feel about prayer? If so, I'm glad you have joined this Bible study! Because I, too, have struggled with prayer. In fact, it's been the biggest fight in my Christian walk. I have constantly seemed to struggle with concentration, content, and consistency. And that's the primary reason the Daniel Prayer has taught me and blessed me and encouraged me and inspired me and motivated me to pray as Daniel prayed!

One key to praying like Daniel is to pray in response to God's Word. It's called "reversed thunder"—praying God's Word back to Him. So I always take my Bible into my prayer time, listening for God's voice to speak to me as I read it. Then I speak . . . or pray . . . back to Him regarding what He has said.

Does this bring up another issue for you? Do you find yourself wishing that God would speak audibly to you like He did with people in the Bible? He spoke to the prophets, the priests, the kings, the elderly, the apostles, the early church, and even to young children like little Samuel. Sometimes, He spoke to the enemies of His people. But whenever He spoke, His voice was so clear to the person listening that there was no mistaking what He had said. How can you hear God's voice today?

While God can speak any way He chooses, He speaks to me through His Word, as He did to Daniel in Daniel 9. In each of the six Bible study sessions, I'm going to lead you in a simple exercise that I use in order to listen to God's voice, which is a springboard into prayer. Then, in each video segment, I will share insights God has given me on that week's topic from Daniel's prayer. Following the video, you will participate in a discussion with your group as you seek ways that Daniel's story and effective prayer life applies to your own.

Commit now to spending time every day in God's Word in order to discover relevant insights for your life that will then become the content for your prayers. This will make each week's discussion time with your group more rewarding, and it will equip you to grow deeper in your faith and more effective in your own prayers. To help you do this, at the end of each session you will be asked to follow Daniel's example by writing out your personal prayers to God.

My prayer for you is that by the end of this study, your own prayers will have become much more vibrant and so effective that Heaven is moved and your world and our nation are changed. For the glory of His great name! So . . . get ready to pray in a way you may never have prayed before. Get ready to pray as Daniel did!

ABOUT THE STUDY

This study guide is to be used with the video-based course *The Daniel Prayer: Prayer That Moves Heaven and Changes Nations.* As an integral part of the course, it provides a format for Bible study that serves as the basis for both small group use (Sunday school classes, women's or men's groups, home or neighborhood studies, one-on-one discipleship) and individual use. This guide will lead you through a series of questions that will enable you to not only discover for yourself the eternal truths revealed by God in the Bible but also to hear God speaking personally to you through His Word. You will then be prepared to participate in a meaningful time of study and discussion with members of your small group.

INDIVIDUAL STUDY

The course begins with a Bible study workshop. After participating in the workshop, you will be familiar with an approach to Bible study that will challenge you to hear and apply God's Word as never before. Beginning in session 2, you will find several portions of Scripture reading to help you apply this method during the course.

> *Note: Each session will require approximately sixty minutes of group meeting time to review the Pre-session Bible study readings, watch the video, discuss the content, and complete the "Choices" exercise. A Simplified and Abbreviated Bible Study plan has been included on pages 115–146 for groups with more limited meeting time, such as in a workplace lunchtime setting.*

It is important to complete each Scripture portion before your next session, as this will make the video presentation more meaningful to you during the small group time. Note that effective daily Bible study will occur if you:

- Set aside a regular place for private devotions.
- Set aside a regular time for private devotions.
- Pray before beginning the day's assignment, asking God to speak to you through His Word.
- Write out your answers for each step in sequence.
- Make the time to be still and listen, reflecting thoughtfully on your response in the final step.
- Don't rush—it may take time in prayerful meditation on a given passage to discover meaningful lessons and hear God speaking to you.

Spiritual discipline is an essential part of your ability to grow in your relationship with God through knowledge and understanding of His Word. So take your individual study seriously and allow God to speak to you from His Word.

GROUP STUDY

In session 1 of *The Daniel Prayer*, you will watch the video workshop and be introduced to this Bible study method. You will be given a passage of Scripture during the workshop to study to help you better understand this approach. At the start of each subsequent session, you will be given some time to share insights from your weekly reading before you and your group watch the video portion. (Note that if your group meets less frequently than once a week, you may want to extend your study time for each passage.)

Space is provided for you to take notes during the video presentation. After the message, you will then have time to discuss the key concepts with your small group using the questions in this guide. (Note that even though there are a number of questions listed for your small group to discuss, you don't need to use them all.

Your leader will focus on the ones that resonate most with your group and guide you from there.)

VIDEO SESSION ACCESS

Streaming video access is included with this study guide. There are streaming video access instructions on how to access all of the video sessions on the inside front cover of this study guide.

Simply go to studygateway.com/redeem to set up your account and enter your access code to add this study to your new Bible study library. Each time you wish to view a video, simply log in to studygateway.com/login and click on the session or study you wish to view. All of your HarperChristian Resources Bible studies with streaming access will be added to your library as you do more studies and redeem the appropriate codes.

INDIVIDUAL COMMITMENT

At the end of the second session, you will be asked to make specific choices as it relates to praying the Daniel Prayer. In subsequent sessions, you will be asked to update your previous choices as you apply any new insights from the current lesson. At the conclusion of the study, you will be encouraged to review these choices as building blocks that have helped you grow in your faith. Your choices will help you develop your personal relationship with God and give you an increasingly richer and more meaningful prayer life.

Remember that the real growth in this study will happen during your quiet times with God during the week. During the group times, you will have the opportunity to process what you have learned with the other members, ask questions, and learn from them as you listen to what God is doing in their lives. In addition, keep in mind that the videos, discussions, and activities in this study are simply meant to sharpen your focus so that you are not only open to what God wants you to hear but also know how to apply that to your life.

> *Note: If you are the facilitator for the group, there are additional instructions and resources provided in the facilitator's guide included in the back of this guide. This separate guide will help you structure your meeting time, facilitate discussion times, and help you lead group members through the key points of the study.*

BIBLE STUDY WORKSHOP

This Bible study workshop has a single purpose: to present an approach that will help you learn to listen for God's voice, know Him in a personal relationship, and communicate with Him through His Word. The following information is introduced in detail in the video presentation. Use this section of the study guide as you view the workshop material. Underline key thoughts and take additional notes as you participate in the workshop. (Note that the passages Anne uses as examples in the video workshop are found on pages 20–23.)

WHAT YOU NEED

Before you begin the video workshop for this first session, you will need the following:

- [ ] a Bible
- [ ] this study guide
- [ ] computer, TV, tablet, or phone for streaming
- [ ] pen or pencil
- [ ] time
- [ ] prayer
- [ ] an open heart

WATCH VIDEO SESSION 1—BIBLE STUDY WORKSHOP (48 MINUTES)

Watch video streaming or on DVD.

Anne will use this video session to walk you through the following five steps to Bible study with the three questions that are essential to the Bible Study Workshop. Anne will illustrate how to do this Bible study with Jonah 1:1-2. (See pages 20-21 in your study guide.)

STEPS TO BIBLE STUDY

STEP 1: READ GOD'S WORD

The first step is *to read the Bible*. At the start of each session in this study guide, you will find the Scriptures listed in a column that you should read during the week. When you have finished reading the passage for the day, move on to step 2.

STEP 2: WHAT DOES GOD'S WORD SAY?
(List the facts.)

After reading the passage, make a verse-by-verse list of the outstanding facts. Don't get caught up in the details—just pinpoint the most obvious facts as they appear to you. When you make your list, do not paraphrase the text but use actual words from the passage. Look for the nouns and the verbs.

STEP 3: WHAT DOES GOD'S WORD MEAN?
(Learn the lessons.)

After reading the passage and listing the facts, look for a lesson to learn from each fact. Ask yourself the following questions:

- *Who is speaking?*
- *What is the subject?*
- *Where is it taking place?*
- *When did it happen?*
- *What can I learn from what is taking place or what is being said?*

  It may also help to ask yourself these questions:

- *What are the people in the passage doing that I should be doing?*
- *Is there a command I should obey?*

- *Is there a promise I should claim?*
- *Is there a warning I should heed?*
- *Is there an example I should follow?*

Focus on spiritual lessons.

STEP 4: WHAT DOES GOD'S WORD MEAN IN MY LIFE? *(Listen to His voice.)*

Although this step will be the most meaningful for you, you can't do it effectively until you complete the first three steps. So, first rephrase the lessons you found in step 3 and put them in the form of questions you could ask yourself, your spouse, your child, your friend, your neighbor, or your coworker. As you write the questions, listen for God to speak to you through His Word.

Be aware that there are some challenging passages in this study. Don't get hung up on what you don't understand, but just look for the *general principles* and *lessons* that can be learned. The introduction prior to the passages you will study in sessions 2–6, as well as the examples offered in steps 2, 3, and 4 of this session, will help you get started.

Remember not to rush this process. It may take you several moments of prayerful meditation to discover meaningful lessons from the Scripture you are reading and hear God speaking to you. The object is not to "get through it" but to develop your personal relationship with God in order to grow in faith and learn to pray in ways that change the world.

STEP 5: HOW WILL I RESPOND TO GOD'S WORD? *(Live it out!)*

Read the assigned Scripture passages prayerfully, objectively, thoughtfully, and attentively as you listen for God to speak. Note that He may not speak to you through *every* verse, but He *will* speak. When He does, record the verse number (if applicable), what it is that God seems to be saying to you, and your response to Him. You might like to date these pages as a means not only of keeping a spiritual journal but also of holding yourself accountable to follow through in obedience. (See pages 20–21 for the example that Anne demonstrates in the video.)

YOUR TURN

Now that you have seen this example from Jonah 1:1–2, it is your turn to try this method on your own using Luke 11:1–4. As you read this passage on pages 22–23, remember to wipe your mind clean of anything others have told you about it or things you have learned before. Keep your mind open, come to the passage looking for fresh insight, and listen for the Lord to speak to you through it.

BIBLE STUDY EXAMPLE

STEP 1

Read God's Word
Passage: Jonah 2:1–2

1 From inside the fish Jonah prayed to the LORD his God.

2 He said: "In my distress I called to the LORD, and he answered me. From the depths of the grave. I called for help, and you listened to my cry."

STEP 2

What Does God's Word Say?
(List the facts.)

v. 1: From inside the fish, Jonah prayed.

v. 1: Jonah prayed to his God.

v. 2: In distress I called to the Lord, and he answered.

v. 2: From the depths of the grave I called for help, and you listened.

STEP 3

What Does God's Word Mean?
(Learn the lessons.)

v. 1: We can pray anywhere.

v. 1: We need to establish a relationship with God <u>before</u> a crisis so we can pray with confidence <u>in a crisis.</u>

v. 2: God responds to our distress calls even when it's our fault that we are in that crisis in the first place.

v. 2: There is no place so low that God doesn't hear our call and cries for help!

STEP 4

What Does God's Word Mean in My Life?
(Listen to His voice.)

v. 1: In what place do I think prayer is off limits?

v. 1: How confident am I in my relationship with God that He will answer me in any situation?

v. 2: Why do I sometimes think that God will not respond to my distress call?

v. 2: If God heard Jonah from the belly of a fish, why don't I think He will hear my call from the depths of depression, addiction, humiliation, or grief?

STEP 5

How Will I Respond to God's Word?
(Live it out!)

Regardless of where I am or what I am going through, I know that God will hear me when I call out to Him. Therefore, I will go to God with confidence, knowing that He will hear and answer me when I seek to pray in ways that move Heaven and change nations.

Name: _____ Date: _____

"YOUR TURN" STUDY

<table>
<tr>
<td>

STEP 1

Read God's Word

Passage: Luke 11:1–4

[1] One day Jesus was praying in a certain place. When he finished, one of his disciples said to him, "Lord, teach us to pray, just as John taught his disciples."

[2] He said to them, "When you pray, say: 'Father, hallowed be your name, your kingdom come.

[3] "'Give us each day our daily bread.

[4] "'Forgive us our sins, for we also forgive everyone who sins against us. And lead us not into temptation.'"

</td>
<td>

STEP 2

What Does God's Word Say?
(List the facts.)

</td>
</tr>
</table>

STEP 3

What Does God's Word Mean?
(Learn the lessons.)

STEP 4

What Does God's Word Mean in My Life?
(Listen to His voice.)

STEP 5

How Will I Respond to God's Word?
(Live it out!)

Name: _____ Date: _____

MOVING FORWARD

For the next session, you will be assigned Matthew 6:5–18 to study using these simple steps you have just learned. This passage has been selected because in it Jesus gives such clear instructions on preparing for prayer, which is the subject of session 2. Make sure to complete the worksheets on pages 28–37 before your next meeting.

> **Note:** *If you are following the Simplified and Abbreviated Bible Study plan, you will be discussing Daniel 6:10 with your group next week. Review the worksheet on pages 118–119 and follow that track for the rest of the study.*

Once you've studied these passages, you will be ready to discuss what you've discovered when you come together with your other group members. Remember that each session of this study is designed to help you follow the steps that Daniel took to pray in ways that move Heaven and change nations. As you go through this course, you will discover how he *prepared* for prayer, was *prompted* in prayer, *pleaded* in prayer, *prevailed* in prayer, and *battled* in prayer. You will learn from Daniel's example how to pray more effectively—and that will make a profound difference in your world today.

PREPARING FOR PRAYER

Just as an athlete can't expect to win by showing up at game time without having practiced, the commitment to pray doesn't just happen. It requires preparation.

Anne Graham Lotz

When we first meet Daniel, we find that he and his people (the Israelites living in Judah) were in trouble. After years of warnings from God to turn from their wicked ways, judgment had finally come upon them in the form of a foreign invading force. "In the third year of the reign of Jehoiakim king of Judah, Nebuchadnezzar king of Babylon came to Jerusalem and besieged it" (Daniel 1:1). In a relatively short period of time, Judah was erased from the map. She no longer existed as she had for more than 500 years. She was a people and a nation in exile.

Daniel was approximately fifteen years of age when he was captured by the Babylonians, taken from his homeland, and transported 800 miles away to serve as a slave in the king's court. In a moment, everything about Daniel's life changed: his culture, his customs, his language, his clothes, and his name. Because his immediate superior was chief of the eunuchs, he may also have been cruelly stripped of his masculinity to make him more subservient to his new master. His situation must have seemed utterly hopeless to him—because, in every obvious way, it was. Yet through it all, Daniel maintained his faith in God and his devotion to Him.

We see this most clearly in the way that Daniel made prayer the center of his life. He never forgot the temple that had been at the heart of Jerusalem and of the nation. Even later in his life, he remained mindful of the sacrifices that had been offered to God there as an act of worship. He longed for Jerusalem every day, as evidenced by the fact that three times daily, when he prayed, he turned his face in the direction of his beloved city that once had been.

Daniel had to make a choice after his circumstances so drastically changed. He could have chosen to be bitter against God. He could have chosen to turn his back on his people. He could have chosen to just compromise with his new culture. But instead, he turned to God and sought to change his people's situation through fervent prayer.

On one occasion, we overhear him pleading with God on behalf of his nation. Ultimately, God answered by moving a ruler named Cyrus to issue a decree that after seventy years of captivity, every Jew living in Babylon could return home. Just think about this. What kind of prayer—offered by one person—could move Heaven and change nations? What was needed for Daniel to be able to pray in that way? What can we learn from his example?

One of the first lessons we learn is that kind of prayer requires *preparation*. The kind of preparation Jesus taught His disciples in Matthew 6.

PRE-SESSION BIBLE STUDY

Begin this week by reading Matthew 6:5–18, and then work through each of the personal Bible studies using the steps you learned in the workshop. You will review the lessons and personal applications during your group session and then watch the teaching from Anne, which points out the application in Daniel's life of the principles Jesus taught.

STUDY 1

STEP 1	**STEP 2**

Read God's Word

Passage: Matthew 6:5

STEP 2

What Does God's Word Say?
(List the facts.)

5 "And when you pray, do not be like the hypocrites, for they love to pray standing in the synagogues and on the street corners to be seen by men. I tell you the truth, they have received their reward in full."

STEP 3

What Does God's Word Mean?
(Learn the lessons.)

STEP 4

What Does God's Word Mean in My Life?
(Listen to His voice.)

STEP 5

How Will I Respond to God's Word?
(Live it out!)

Name: _____ Date: _____

STUDY 2

STEP 1

Read God's Word

Passage: Matthew 6:6

6 "But when you pray, go into your room, close the door and pray to your Father, who is unseen. Then your Father, who sees what is done in secret, will reward you."

STEP 2

What Does God's Word Say?

(List the facts.)

STEP 3

What Does God's Word Mean?
(Learn the lessons.)

STEP 4

What Does God's Word Mean in My Life?
(Listen to His voice.)

STEP 5

How Will I Respond to God's Word?
(Live it out!)

Name: _____ Date: _____

STUDY 3

STEP 1	STEP 2
Read God's Word	*What Does God's Word Say?*
Passage: Matthew 6:7–8	*(List the facts.)*

7 "And when you pray, do not keep on babbling like pagans, for they think they will be heard because of their many words.

8 "Do not be like them, for your Father knows what you need before you ask him."

STEP 3

What Does God's Word Mean?
(Learn the lessons.)

STEP 4

What Does God's Word Mean in My Life?
(Listen to His voice.)

STEP 5

How Will I Respond to God's Word?
(Live it out!)

Name: _____ Date: _____

STUDY 4

STEP 1	STEP 2
Read God's Word	*What Does God's Word Say?*
Passage: Matthew 6:9–13	*(List the facts.)*

9 "This, then, is how you should pray: 'Our Father in heaven, hallowed be your name,

10 "'your kingdom come, your will be done on earth as it is in heaven.

11 "'Give us today our daily bread.

12 "'Forgive us our debts, as we also have forgiven our debtors.

13 "'And lead us not into temptation, but deliver us from the evil one.'"

STEP 3

What Does God's Word Mean?
(Learn the lessons.)

STEP 4

What Does God's Word Mean in My Life?
(Listen to His voice.)

STEP 5

How Will I Respond to God's Word?
(Live it out!)

Name: _____ Date: _____

STUDY 5

STEP 1

Read God's Word
Passage: Matthew 6:14–18

14 "For if you forgive men when they sin against you, your heavenly Father will also forgive you.

15 "But if you do not forgive men their sins, your Father will not forgive your sins.

16 "When you fast, do not look somber as the hypocrites do, for they disfigure their faces to show men they are fasting. I tell you the truth, they have received their reward in full.

17 "But when you fast, put oil on your head and wash your face,

18 "so that it will not be obvious to men that you are fasting, but only to your Father, who is unseen; and your Father, who sees what is done in secret, will reward you."

STEP 2

What Does God's Word Say?
(List the facts.)

STEP 3

What Does God's Word Mean?
(Learn the lessons.)

STEP 4

What Does God's Word Mean in My Life?
(Listen to His voice.)

STEP 5

How Will I Respond to God's Word?
(Live it out!)

Name: _____ Date: _____

WATCH VIDEO SESSION 2—
PREPARING FOR PRAYER

Watch video streaming or on DVD.

Use this space to take notes if you like:

GROUP DISCUSSION QUESTIONS

Open your group discussion sharing something in the video teaching that was either striking or was new to you altogether.

1. What is the "Daniel Prayer"? How is it different from other kinds of prayer?

2. What is the best place for you to meet God each day in prayer? Share your ideas, settle on the best one for you, and commit to do it.

3. What is the best time for you to set aside for prayer?

4. How can you create an atmosphere that is more conducive for prayer?

5. What are some ways you can cultivate an attitude of gratitude when you come to God in prayer?

CHOICES

This week, you studied Matthew 6:5–18 and learned what Jesus teaches about preparing for prayer. Think back on how you responded to this passage of Scripture (step 5 in your daily studies). Write down some areas you need to work on to better prepare your heart to pray as Daniel did.

What I will do to prepare for prayer . . .

WRAPPING UP

Some 700 years before the conquest of Judah, King Solomon had prayed, "When [the people] sin against you . . . and you become angry with them and give them over to the enemy . . . and if they turn back to you with all their heart and soul in the land of their enemies who took them captive, and pray to you toward the land you gave their fathers . . . then from heaven, your dwelling place, hear their prayer and their plea" (1 Kings 8:46, 48–49). Daniel had followed this practice of praying toward Jerusalem during his captivity, and he did not alter it even in the face of death. Why was he so committed to this practice?

> *Three times a day, when Daniel went to his designated place for prayer, he opened his windows toward Jerusalem. The poignant gesture revealed not only the longing in his heart for his city and his people, but also his exclusive focus on the God of Abraham, Isaac, and Jacob. The God of his fathers. The God who had been with him throughout his lifetime, for over eighty years. The one, true, living God whom Daniel worshiped and served and obeyed.*
>
> —Anne Graham Lotz, *The Daniel Prayer*, page 38

Daniel had cultivated a lifetime habit of prayer and was unwilling to compromise even the smallest detail in his worship to the Lord. Even though he was in captivity and under constant threat, three times a day—without fail—he expressed his thankfulness to God. Today, as you prepare to move forward, consider what it would look like for you to cultivate such an attitude toward God. On the lines provided, write out your own heart-prayer to God, expressing your gratitude to Him in spite of whatever challenges or trials you are facing.

MY PRAYER

_____

_____

_____

_____

_____

_____

_____

_____

_____

_____

_____

MOVING FORWARD

For the next session, you will be assigned 2 Chronicles 6:40–7:22 to study using the approach you learned in the Bible study workshop. Make sure to complete the worksheets on pages 46–55 before your next meeting. Once you take the first step of preparing a time, place, atmosphere, and attitude for prayer, you are ready for the next step. You must now consider what *prompts* you to pray the kind of heartfelt cry to God that Daniel prayed for others. We will examine this aspect of the Daniel Prayer in the next session.

PROMPTING IN PRAYER

The Daniel Prayer is not just venting to God. . . . It is an outpouring of heartfelt emotion and passionate pleading based on God's Word as we hold Him to His promises.

Anne Graham Lotz

Are you intimidated by prayer? Have you ever prayed simply because it was expected of you? Maybe you've encountered this in your small group. Everyone is praying around the circle, and you feel you have no way of getting out of it. All the while, as people are praying, you're thinking about what in the world you are going to say when it's your turn.

Maybe this has conditioned you to pray in certain ways about certain things just to be polite. You pray for your children. Or for your friends at church. Or for the missionaries in Africa and other faraway places. As you do, you try your best not to stutter or lose your train of thought for fear of sounding silly. Perhaps this type of conditioning has left you feeling that prayer is just a chore. Overall, it seems pretty useless in your life.

Perhaps you are wondering what it would take for you to pray in the way that Daniel prayed. After all, as we have seen, there was nothing professional or formulaic about his conversations with God. He didn't pray out of obligation or to be polite in the presence of others. No, he was *compelled* to pray passionate, heartfelt, laser-focused, soul-gripping prayers until the very throne of Heaven was moved. What was his secret?

Daniel knew his world had problems. He knew his people had problems. He knew *he* had problems. As we noted in the last session, by the time he prayed in Daniel 9, he was an old man. He had seen not only the demise of Judah at the hands of the Babylonians, but also the demise of Babylon at the hands of the Medes and Persians. His position was precarious and uncertain under the new rulers. He was living in an unsettled and changing world.

So, when Daniel came across a promise in Scripture that God would bring His people back from captivity after seventy years (see Jeremiah 29:10), he was *prompted* to claim that promise. He based his prayer on God's Word and basically said it back to the Lord. He "reversed the thunder," as Eugene Peterson says, and held God to His Word.

Apply this to your life. As you look at your world today, what problems do you see? How are those problems compelling you to pray? Are you basing your prayers on what you want or hope—or on the promises of God? The Lord has said, "if my people, who are called by my name, will humble themselves and pray and seek my face and turn from their wicked ways, then will I hear from heaven and will forgive their sin and will heal their land" (2 Chronicles 7:14). How can you and I claim this promise as we hold God to it?

In this week's Bible study, we will once again go outside the book of Daniel to a dramatic scene from 2 Chronicles. King David's son Solomon had built a magnificent temple for God in Jerusalem. Our passage opens with Solomon publicly dedicating it to God and invoking His presence, and it concludes with God's public and private response to Solomon. As you read, look for what God told Solomon should prompt his prayers for his nation—and how that should prompt ours as well, so that we pray as Daniel did.

PRE-SESSION BIBLE STUDY

Begin this week by reading 2 Chronicles 6:40–7:22, and then work through each of the personal Bible studies using the steps you learned in the workshop. You will review the lessons and personal applications during your group session and then watch the teaching from Anne.

STUDY 1

STEP 1

Read God's Word

Passage: 2 Chronicles 6:40–42

40 "Now, my God, may your eyes be open and your ears attentive to the prayers offered in this place.

41 "Now arise, O Lord God, and come to your resting place, you and the ark of your might. May your priests, O Lord God, be clothed with salvation, may your saints rejoice in your goodness.

42 "O Lord, do not reject your anointed one. Remember the great love promised to David your servant."

STEP 2

What Does God's Word Say?

(List the facts.)

STEP 3

What Does God's Word Mean?
(Learn the lessons.)

STEP 4

What Does God's Word Mean in My Life?
(Listen to His voice.)

STEP 5

How Will I Respond to God's Word?
(Live it out!)

Name: _____ Date: _____

STEP 1

Read God's Word

Passage: 2 Chronicles 7:1–6

¹ When Solomon finished praying, fire came down from heaven and consumed the burnt offering and the sacrifices, and the glory of the LORD filled the temple.

² The priests could not enter the temple of the LORD because the glory of the LORD filled it.

³ When all the Israelites saw the fire coming down and the glory of the LORD above the temple, they knelt on the pavement with their faces to the ground, and they worshiped and gave thanks to the LORD, saying, "He is good; his love endures forever."

⁴ Then the king and all the people offered sacrifices before the LORD.

⁵ And King Solomon offered a sacrifice of twenty-two thousand head of cattle and a hundred and twenty thousand sheep and goats. So the king and all the people dedicated the temple of God.

⁶ The priests took their positions, as did the Levites with the LORD's musical instruments, which King David had made for praising the LORD and which were used when he gave thanks, saying, "His love endures forever." Opposite the Levites, the priests blew their trumpets, and all the Israelites were standing.

STEP 2

What Does God's Word Say?
(List the facts.)

STEP 3

What Does God's Word Mean?
(Learn the lessons.)

STEP 4

What Does God's Word Mean in My Life?
(Listen to His voice.)

STEP 5

How Will I Respond to God's Word?
(Live it out!)

Name: _____ Date: _____

STEP 1

Read God's Word

Passage: 2 Chronicles 7:7–10

⁷ Solomon consecrated the middle part of the courtyard in front of the temple of the LORD, and there he offered burnt offerings and the fat of the fellowship offerings, because the bronze altar he had made could not hold the burnt offerings, the grain offerings and the fat portions.

⁸ So Solomon observed the festival at that time for seven days, and all Israel with him—a vast assembly, people from Lebo Hamath to the Wadi of Egypt.

⁹ On the eighth day they held an assembly, for they had celebrated the dedication of the altar for seven days and the festival for seven days more.

¹⁰ On the twenty-third day of the seventh month he sent the people to their homes, joyful and glad in heart for the good things the LORD had done for David and Solomon and for his people Israel.

STEP 2

What Does God's Word Say?

(List the facts.)

STEP 3

What Does God's Word Mean?
(Learn the lessons.)

STEP 4

What Does God's Word Mean in My Life?
(Listen to His voice.)

STEP 5

How Will I Respond to God's Word?
(Live it out!)

Name: _____ Date: _____

STEP 1

Read God's Word
Passage: 2 Chronicles 7:11–16

11 When Solomon had finished the temple of the LORD and the royal palace, and had succeeded in carrying out all he had in mind to do in the temple of the LORD and in his own palace,

12 the LORD appeared to him at night and said: "I have heard your prayer and have chosen this place for myself as a temple for sacrifices.

13 "When I shut up the heavens so that there is no rain, or command locusts to devour the land or send a plague among my people,

14 "if my people, who are called by my name, will humble themselves and pray and seek my face and turn from their wicked ways, then will I hear from heaven and will forgive their sin and will heal their land.

15 "Now my eyes will be open and my ears attentive to the prayers offered in this place.

16 "I have chosen and consecrated this temple so that my Name may be there forever. My eyes and my heart will always be there."

STEP 2

What Does God's Word Say?
(List the facts.)

STEP 3

What Does God's Word Mean?
(Learn the lessons.)

STEP 4

What Does God's Word Mean in My Life?
(Listen to His voice.)

STEP 5

How Will I Respond to God's Word?
(Live it out!)

Name: _____ Date: _____

STUDY 5

Read God's Word

Passage: 2 Chronicles 7:17–22

What Does God's Word Say?
(List the facts.)

17 "As for you, if you walk before me as David your father did, and do all I command, and observe my decrees and laws,

18 "I will establish your royal throne, as I covenanted with David your father when I said, 'You shall never fail to have a man to rule over Israel.'

19 "But if you turn away and forsake the decrees and commands I have given you and go off to serve other gods and worship them,

20 "then I will uproot Israel from my land, which I have given them, and will reject this temple I have consecrated for my Name. I will make it a byword and an object of ridicule among all peoples.

21 "And though this temple is now so imposing, all who pass by will be appalled and say, 'Why has the LORD done such a thing to this land and to this temple?'

22 "People will answer, 'Because they have forsaken the LORD, the God of their fathers, who brought them out of Egypt, and have embraced other gods, worshiping and serving them—that is why he brought all this disaster on them.'"

STEP 3

What Does God's Word Mean?
(Learn the lessons.)

STEP 4

What Does God's Word Mean in My Life?
(Listen to His voice.)

STEP 5

How Will I Respond to God's Word?
(Live it out!)

Name: _____ Date: _____

WATCH VIDEO SESSION 3—
PROMPTING IN PRAYER

Watch video streaming or on DVD.

Use this space to take notes if you like:

GROUP DISCUSSION QUESTIONS

Open your group discussion sharing something in the video teaching that was either striking or was new to you altogether.

1. What situations in your life or in the world have motivated you to pray?

2. What are some promises God has given to you in His Word that you have claimed relating to the above situation?

3. What does it mean to "hold God to His Word" in prayer?

4. What helps you to stay centered on God when you pray?

5. How does humility play a part in praying the Daniel Prayer?

CHOICES

This week, you studied Solomon's experience in 2 Chronicles 6:40–7:22 as God instructed him in how to pray when disaster strikes or troubles come. Think back on how you responded to this passage of Scripture (step 5 in your daily studies). Write down some areas you need to work on or incorporate personally. Then, go back to your choices from the last session. Is there anything you now want to add or delete? Is there any further insight or additional choice you want to make? If so, write it below.

What I will do to pray under compulsion . . .

WRAPPING UP

If you've ever been lost, you know the value of having a GPS. All you need to do is type in the location of where you want to go, and the GPS will provide directions for how to get there. As long as you are focused on following those directions, you will find your way home. The same is true of prayer. All you need to do when you are lost is to go to God, and He will provide the directions. But you have to focus on *following* those directions to find your way home.

> *[God] is the Center-point. When our prayers are focused, regardless of what life throws at us, whether it's a long, hard climb to the top of our profession or career, or the steady trail of perseverance as we set out to achieve our goals, or the confusion and lost feeling that can envelop us when we find ourselves in a thicket of problems and pressures and pain—if our prayers are focused on the living God, they will make a difference.*

—Anne Graham Lotz, *The Daniel Prayer*, page 65

Daniel had this type of laser-focus when he responded to the promptings he felt to pray for God's people. Before he spoke even a word, he "turned to the LORD God" (Daniel 9:3). The Lord was his Center-point, and regardless of the situation, he knew that God would deliver on His promises. Today, consider what would prompt you to pray as Daniel prayed. What would it look like for you to center on God privately, sincerely, desperately, and humbly? What promises from the Bible do you need God to bring to mind? On the lines below, write out your own heart-prayer to God in response to these questions.

MY PRAYER

_____

_____

_____

_____

_____

_____

_____

_____

_____

_____

_____

_____

_____

MOVING FORWARD

For the next session, you will be assigned Nehemiah 1:1–2:9 to study using the approach you learned in the Bible study workshop. This passage focuses on what it means to plead in prayer, which is the topic for our study. Make sure to complete the worksheets on pages 64–73 before your next meeting. Once you consider what compels you to pray and how you should be centered on God when you pray, you are ready for the next step. You should now consider what it looks like to *plead* in prayer as Daniel did for his people. We will examine this aspect of the Daniel Prayer in the next session.

PLEADING IN PRAYER

Daniel was confident of who God was. He knew God belonged to him and that he belonged to God. This covenant relationship with God was the bedrock of the Daniel Prayer.

Anne Graham Lotz

When you turn to God in prayer, do you ever feel disconnected from Him? Maybe you feel a bit like Dorothy in *The Wizard of Oz* when she spoke with the ruler of the Emerald City. She thought she was meeting a mighty and powerful wizard, but when the curtain was pulled back, he ended up just being an ordinary man from Omaha. The wizard was not at all what Dorothy expected. And he was nothing like what she needed at that moment.

For Daniel to plead with God in the way he did, he had to have confidence in God's *character*—in His faithfulness, righteousness, goodness, and greatness. He had to believe the Lord was who He said He was and that He actually had the power to help him. Daniel also had to have confidence in his *relationship* with God. He had to be in a place where he knew that he could plead with the Lord in prayer, and the Lord would answer him. Daniel had to be in a covenant relationship with the Lord to pray as he did.

A *covenant* is a legal agreement between two or more parties, as in a treaty or formal agreement between nations, or a land covenant between the buyer and the seller of property. Daniel knew this form of covenant relationship with God was vitally important in prayer. The Lord can answer any prayer He chooses, but Daniel knew that when he entered into a covenant relationship with God, he was *guaranteed* to receive an answer.

The same is true for us today. God promises in His Word that "if we confess our sins, he is faithful and just and will forgive us our sins and purify us from all unrighteousness" (1 John 1:9). If we confess our sins (contrition), put our faith in God's Word, and believe, we are assured that God will forgive us. This gives us the confidence to then pray the words of the Daniel Prayer as we plead for God to move in our world.

In this week's Bible study, our passage is from Nehemiah, another great Old Testament leader. Like Daniel, he was an Israelite enslaved in Babylon, living in exile as the cupbearer to the king. He received a very disturbing report concerning Jerusalem, and our passage examines his response. Look for the words he prayed that demonstrated his knowledge of God's *character* and the type of *relationship* that he had with the Lord. Also look for how Nehemiah pleaded with *contrition* (confessing sins) and *clarity*.

PRE-SESSION BIBLE STUDY

Begin this week by reading Nehemiah 1:1–2:9, and then work through each of the personal Bible studies using the steps you learned in the workshop. You will review the lessons and personal applications during your group session and then watch the teaching from Anne.

STUDY 1

STEP 1	STEP 2
Read God's Word	*What Does God's Word Say?*
Passage: Nehemiah 1:1–3	*(List the facts.)*

1 The words of Nehemiah son of Hacaliah: In the month of Kislev in the twentieth year, while I was in the citadel of Susa,

2 Hanani, one of my brothers, came from Judah with some other men, and I questioned them about the Jewish remnant that survived the exile, and also about Jerusalem.

3 They said to me, "Those who survived the exile and are back in the province are in great trouble and disgrace. The wall of Jerusalem is broken down, and its gates have been burned with fire."

STEP 3

What Does God's Word Mean?
(Learn the lessons.)

STEP 4

What Does God's Word Mean in My Life?
(Listen to His voice.)

STEP 5

How Will I Respond to God's Word?
(Live it out!)

Name: _____ Date: _____

STEP 1

Read God's Word

Passage: Nehemiah 1:4–11

4 When I heard these things, I sat down and wept. For some days I mourned and fasted and prayed before the God of heaven.

5 Then I said: "O Lord, God of heaven, the great and awesome God, who keeps his covenant of love with those who love him and obey his commands,

6 "let your ear be attentive and your eyes open to hear the prayer your servant is praying before you day and night for your servants, the people of Israel. I confess the sins we Israelites, including myself and my father's house, have committed against you.

7 "We have acted very wickedly toward you. We have not obeyed the commands, decrees and laws you gave your servant Moses.

8 "Remember the instruction you gave your servant Moses, saying, 'If you are unfaithful, I will scatter you among the nations,

9 "'but if you return to me and obey my commands, then even if your exiled people are at the farthest horizon, I will gather them from there and bring them to the place I have chosen as a dwelling for my Name.'

10 "They are your servants and your people, whom you redeemed by your great strength and your mighty hand.

11 "O Lord, let your ear be attentive to the prayer of this your servant and to the prayer of your servants who delight in revering your name. Give your servant success today by granting him favor in the presence of this man." I was cupbearer to the king.

STEP 2

What Does God's Word Say?

(List the facts.)

STEP 3

What Does God's Word Mean?
(Learn the lessons.)

STEP 4

What Does God's Word Mean in My Life?
(Listen to His voice.)

STEP 5

How Will I Respond to God's Word?
(Live it out!)

Name: _____ Date: _____

STEP 1

Read God's Word

Passage: Nehemiah 2:1–3

1 In the month of Nisan in the twentieth year of King Artaxerxes, when wine was brought for him, I took the wine and gave it to the king. I had not been sad in his presence before;

2 so the king asked me, "Why does your face look so sad when you are not ill? This can be nothing but sadness of heart." I was very much afraid,

3 but I said to the king, "May the king live forever! Why should my face not look sad when the city where my fathers are buried lies in ruins, and its gates have been destroyed by fire?"

STEP 2

What Does God's Word Say?

(List the facts.)

STEP 3

What Does God's Word Mean?
(Learn the lessons.)

STEP 4

What Does God's Word Mean in My Life?
(Listen to His voice.)

STEP 5

How Will I Respond to God's Word?
(Live it out!)

Name: _____ Date: _____

STUDY 4

STEP 1	STEP 2
Read God's Word	*What Does God's Word Say?*
Passage: Nehemiah 2:4–6	*(List the facts.)*

⁴ The king said to me, "What is it you want?" Then I prayed to the God of heaven,

⁵ and I answered the king, "If it pleases the king and if your servant has found favor in his sight, let him send me to the city in Judah where my fathers are buried so that I can rebuild it."

⁶ Then the king, with the queen sitting beside him, asked me, "How long will your journey take, and when will you get back?" It pleased the king to send me; so I set a time.

STEP 3

What Does God's Word Mean?
(Learn the lessons.)

STEP 4

What Does God's Word Mean in My Life?
(Listen to His voice.)

STEP 5

How Will I Respond to God's Word?
(Live it out!)

Name: _____ Date: _____

STUDY 5

STEP 1	STEP 2
Read God's Word	*What Does God's Word Say?*
Passage: Nehemiah 2:7–9	*(List the facts.)*

7 I also said to him, "If it pleases the king, may I have letters to the governors of Trans-Euphrates, so that they will provide me safe-conduct until I arrive in Judah?

8 "And may I have a letter to Asaph, keeper of the king's forest, so he will give me timber to make beams for the gates of the citadel by the temple and for the city wall and for the residence I will occupy?" And because the gracious hand of my God was upon me, the king granted my requests.

9 So I went to the governors of Trans-Euphrates and gave them the king's letters. The king had also sent army officers and cavalry with me.

STEP 3

What Does God's Word Mean?
(Learn the lessons.)

STEP 4

What Does God's Word Mean in My Life?
(Listen to His voice.)

STEP 5

How Will I Respond to God's Word?
(Live it out!)

Name: _____ Date: _____

WATCH VIDEO SESSION 4—
PLEADING IN PRAYER

Watch video streaming or on DVD.

Use this space to take notes if you like:

GROUP DISCUSSION QUESTIONS

Open your group discussion sharing something in the video teaching that was either striking or was new to you altogether.

1. What are some of the ways you can build your confidence in God?

2. When was a time God demonstrated His faithfulness and/or His goodness to you? Describe it for the group.

3. When was a time God demonstrated His righteousness and/or His greatness to you? Describe it for the group.

4. What are you asking God for? Pinpoint it with clarity, and share it with your group.

CHOICES

This week, you studied Nehemiah 1:1–2:9 and saw how Nehemiah confessed sin as he pleaded with God to intervene on behalf of Jerusalem. Think back on how you responded to this passage of Scripture (step 5 in your daily studies). Turn the page and write down some areas you need to work on as it relates to examining your own heart as Daniel did in his prayer.

What I will do with what I discover as I examine my heart . . .

WRAPPING UP

In Psalm 51:17, King David wrote, "The sacrifices of God are a broken spirit; a broken and contrite heart, O God, you will not despise." When we pray with contrition—not pointing the finger at others but looking at our own behavior—the Lord assures us that He will accept that kind of approach. Given this, why is it so hard for us to look at the sin in our hearts?

> *I think one reason some of us, myself included, don't examine our hearts for sin is because we are so afraid we will find it. One thing I have discovered is that it takes courage to look deep within to see what God sees. It's painful to acknowledge that we're not as good, righteous, pure, or holy as we thought.*
>
> —Anne Graham Lotz, *The Daniel Prayer*, pages 129–130

Before you apply the Daniel Prayer to the sins of others, it is important to take a moment to look at the sins in your own life. Would you be courageous enough, after reading three times through the list of sins included in the back of this study guide (pages 147–149), to take pen in hand and write out a prayer to God confessing your sins? On the lines below, write out your own heart-prayer to God expressing your sorrow and asking for His forgiveness.

MY PRAYER

_____

_____

_____

_____

_____

_____

_____

_____

_____

_____

_____

MOVING FORWARD

For the next session, you will be assigned 2 Chronicles 20:1–30 to study using the approach you learned in the Bible study workshop. Make sure to complete the worksheets on pages 82–91 before your next meeting. Once you have examined your understanding of God and your relationship with Him, and have confessed your own sins with clarity, you are ready for the next step. You will now consider what is required to *prevail* in prayer until you receive an answer from God. We will examine this aspect of the Daniel Prayer in the next session.

PREVAILING IN PRAYER

Drive the stake of your faith deep down into God's promises. Don't quit. Don't give up. Don't give in. Don't collapse. Don't settle for less than prayer that moves Heaven and changes nations.

Anne Graham Lotz

One day when Jesus was teaching the people, He told them a parable about a persistent widow. The woman had been wronged, and she was determined to get justice. Unfortunately, the judge in the town "neither feared God nor cared about men" (Luke 18:2). For a time, he refused to listen to her. But the woman was so persistent that eventually the judge was forced to say, "Because this widow keeps bothering me, I will see that she gets justice" (verse 5).

Jesus' purpose in telling the story was to show His followers that they should never give up when it comes to prayer. He concluded, "Will not God bring about justice for his chosen ones, who cry out to him day and night? . . . He will see that they get justice, and quickly" (verses 7–8). This is what it means to *prevail* in prayer. It means to just keep on praying . . . and praying . . . *and praying* . . . until God answers.

This doesn't necessarily mean that you stay in a place of prayer 24/7 and refuse to move from that spot. It doesn't mean repeating the exact same prayer over and over because you fear that God has not heard you. What prevailing in prayer does mean is holding a position of prayer in your spirit until you receive the answer. It means wrapping your heart and mind around whatever it is you are asking of God until He responds. It means sticking with the prayer and not just walking away from it when you get discouraged.

God's purpose for having you prevail in prayer is for your own benefit. He looks on the heart of the one who is praying and is moved by that person's trust in Him. He is not an "add-on God"—when you pray, you can't be holding on to some other options that you are relying on just in case God doesn't come through for you. You can't have a Plan A, and if that doesn't work a Plan B, and then only tack on prayer as a last-ditch emergency strategy. God wants you to go to Him first and rely on Him completely. As you prevail in prayer and see Him miraculously provide time and again, it builds your faith and trust in Him.

In previous weeks, we have seen how Daniel established a lifetime habit of persisting in prayer. In this week's Bible study, we are once again going to go outside the book of Daniel and read of another Old Testament leader who dramatically prevailed in prayer. Jehoshaphat was king of Israel when the enemy came against him, and he was faced with an overwhelming and impossible situation. As you study this passage, look for how Jehoshaphat responded to the news of impending disaster, and then how God responded.

PRE-SESSION BIBLE STUDY

Begin this week by reading 2 Chronicles 20:1–30, and then work through each of the personal Bible studies using the steps you learned in the workshop. You will review the lessons and personal applications during your group session and then watch the teaching from Anne.

STUDY 1

STEP 1	STEP 2

STEP 1

Read God's Word

Passage: 2 Chronicles 20:1–4

¹ After this, the Moabites and Ammonites with some of the Meunites came to make war on Jehoshaphat.

² Some men came and told Jehoshaphat, "A vast army is coming against you from Edom, from the other side of the Sea. It is already in Hazazon Tamar" (that is, En Gedi).

³ Alarmed, Jehoshaphat resolved to inquire of the LORD, and he proclaimed a fast for all Judah.

⁴ The people of Judah came together to seek help from the LORD; indeed, they came from every town in Judah to seek him.

STEP 2

What Does God's Word Say?

(List the facts.)

STEP 3

What Does God's Word Mean?
(Learn the lessons.)

STEP 4

What Does God's Word Mean in My Life?
(Listen to His voice.)

STEP 5

How Will I Respond to God's Word?
(Live it out!)

Name: _____ Date: _____

STUDY 2

STEP 1	STEP 2
Read God's Word	*What Does God's Word Say?*
Passage: 2 Chronicles 20:5–12	*(List the facts.)*

5 Then Jehoshaphat stood up in the assembly of Judah and Jerusalem at the temple of the LORD in the front of the new courtyard

6 and said: "O LORD, God of our fathers, are you not the God who is in heaven? You rule over all the kingdoms of the nations. Power and might are in your hand, and no one can withstand you.

7 "O our God, did you not drive out the inhabitants of this land before your people Israel and give it forever to the descendants of Abraham your friend?

8 "They have lived in it and have built in it a sanctuary for your Name, saying,

9 "'If calamity comes upon us, whether the sword of judgment, or plague or famine, we will stand in your presence before this temple that bears your Name and will cry out to you in our distress, and you will hear us and save us.'

10 "But now here are men from Ammon, Moab and Mount Seir, whose territory you would not allow Israel to invade when they came from Egypt; so they turned away from them and did not destroy them.

11 "See how they are repaying us by coming to drive us out of the possession you gave us as an inheritance.

12 "O our God, will you not judge them? For we have no power to face this vast army that is attacking us. We do not know what to do, but our eyes are upon you."

STEP 3
What Does God's Word Mean?
(Learn the lessons.)

STEP 4
What Does God's Word Mean in My Life?
(Listen to His voice.)

STEP 5

How Will I Respond to God's Word?
(Live it out!)

Name: _____ Date: _____

STUDY 3

<table>
<tr><td>

STEP 1

Read God's Word

Passage: 2 Chronicles 20:13–19

</td><td>

STEP 2

What Does God's Word Say?

(List the facts.)

</td></tr>
</table>

13 All the men of Judah, with their wives and children and little ones, stood there before the LORD.

14 Then the Spirit of the LORD came upon Jahaziel son of Zechariah, the son of Benaiah, the son of Jeiel, the son of Mattaniah, a Levite and descendant of Asaph, as he stood in the assembly.

15 He said: "Listen, King Jehoshaphat and all who live in Judah and Jerusalem! This is what the LORD says to you: 'Do not be afraid or discouraged because of this vast army. For the battle is not yours, but God's.

16 "Tomorrow march down against them. They will be climbing up by the Pass of Ziz, and you will find them at the end of the gorge in the Desert of Jeruel.

17 "You will not have to fight this battle. Take up your positions; stand firm and see the deliverance the LORD will give you, O Judah and Jerusalem. Do not be afraid; do not be discouraged. Go out to face them tomorrow, and the LORD will be with you.'"

18 Jehoshaphat bowed with his face to the ground, and all the people of Judah and Jerusalem fell down in worship before the LORD.

19 Then some Levites from the Kohathites and Korahites stood up and praised the LORD, the God of Israel, with very loud voice.

STEP 3

What Does God's Word Mean?
(Learn the lessons.)

STEP 4

What Does God's Word Mean in My Life?
(Listen to His voice.)

STEP 5

How Will I Respond to God's Word?
(Live it out!)

Name: _____ Date: _____

STUDY 4

STEP 1	STEP 2
Read God's Word	*What Does God's Word Say?*
Passage: 2 Chronicles 20:20–23	*(List the facts.)*

20 Early in the morning they left for the Desert of Tekoa. As they set out, Jehoshaphat stood and said, "Listen to me, Judah and people of Jerusalem! Have faith in the LORD your God and you will be upheld; have faith in his prophets and you will be successful."

21 After consulting the people, Jehoshaphat appointed men to sing to the LORD and to praise him for the splendor of his holiness as they went out at the head of the army, saying: "Give thanks to the LORD, for his love endures forever."

22 As they began to sing and praise, the LORD set ambushes against the men of Ammon and Moab and Mount Seir who were invading Judah, and they were defeated.

23 The men of Ammon and Moab rose up against the men from Mount Seir to destroy and annihilate them. After they finished slaughtering the men from Seir, they helped to destroy one another.

STEP 3

What Does God's Word Mean?
(Learn the lessons.)

STEP 4

What Does God's Word Mean in My Life?
(Listen to His voice.)

STEP 5

How Will I Respond to God's Word?
(Live it out!)

Name: _____ Date: _____

STEP 1

Read God's Word

Passage: 2 Chronicles 20:24–30

24 When the men of Judah came to the place that overlooks the desert and looked toward the vast army, they saw only dead bodies lying on the ground; no one had escaped.

25 So Jehoshaphat and his men went to carry off their plunder, and they found among them a great amount of equipment and clothing and also articles of value—more than they could take away. There was so much plunder that it took three days to collect it.

26 On the fourth day they assembled in the Valley of Beracah, where they praised the LORD. This is why it is called the Valley of Beracah to this day.

27 Then, led by Jehoshaphat, all the men of Judah and Jerusalem returned joyfully to Jerusalem, for the LORD had given them cause to rejoice over their enemies.

28 They entered Jerusalem and went to the temple of the LORD with harps and lutes and trumpets.

29 The fear of God came upon all the kingdoms of the countries when they heard how the LORD had fought against the enemies of Israel.

30 And the kingdom of Jehoshaphat was at peace, for his God had given him rest on every side.

STEP 2

What Does God's Word Say?

(List the facts.)

STEP 3

What Does God's Word Mean?
(Learn the lessons.)

STEP 4

What Does God's Word Mean in My Life?
(Listen to His voice.)

STEP 5

How Will I Respond to God's Word?
(Live it out!)

Name: _____ Date: _____

THE DANIEL PRAYER STUDY GUIDE

WATCH VIDEO SESSION 5—
PREVAILING IN PRAYER

Watch video streaming or on DVD.

Use this space to take notes if you like:

GROUP DISCUSSION QUESTIONS

Open your group discussion sharing something in the video teaching that was either striking or was new to you altogether.

1. What does it mean to you personally to prevail in prayer?

2. What are some ways that you have seen God answer your prayers immediately?

3. How has God answered your prayer ultimately? How long did you seek God in prayer before the answer came to you?

4. In what situations have you seen God answer prayer specifically?

5. What helps you not to be discouraged and give up when prevailing in prayer?

CHOICES

This week, you studied 2 Chronicles 20:1–30 and saw how God responded to Jehoshaphat's plea for the Lord to rescue His people and return them to their home-land. Think back on how you responded to this passage of Scripture (step 5 in your daily studies). Write down some areas you need to work on as it relates to prevailing in prayer.

What I will do to prevail in prayer . . .

WRAPPING UP

Jesus gave His disciples many specific instructions on prayer. They were not to pray like the hypocrites who loved to stand out and be noticed by others for their "super spirituality." They were not to go on babbling, as if trying to impress God and others with their words. Instead, they were to simply say, "Your kingdom come, your will be done on earth as it is in heaven" (Matthew 6:10). What does it mean to prevail in prayer for God's will to be done?

> *To prevail in prayer . . . [is] to put your arms of faith about your Father's neck and cling tightly to Him until He blesses you. But to prevail, you must be sure that what you are praying for is something you know God wants to give you. And how do you know what He wants to give you? You base your prayer on God's Word. Then you hold Him to it through prevailing prayer.*
>
> —Anne Graham Lotz, *The Daniel Prayer*, page 172

Remember that when Daniel made his request to God, he was praying back a promise the Lord had already made in the Scriptures. Daniel could approach God confidently because he knew that he was praying for something that God already wanted to give. His act of prevailing in prayer was a means by which he was holding God accountable to His Word. Today, consider what it would look like for you to pray in the same way. On the lines on the next page, write out your own heart-prayer to God based on the promises you have discovered in God's Word.

MY PRAYER

_____

_____

_____

_____

_____

_____

_____

_____

_____

_____

MOVING FORWARD

For the next session, you will be assigned Ephesians 6:10–20 to study using the approach you learned in the Bible study workshop. Make sure to complete the worksheets on pages 100–109 before your next meeting. When you pray the Daniel Prayer, you may receive an immediate answer to your request. However, there will be times when prevailing in prayer doesn't lead to an instantaneous response. In the final session of this study, we will examine another episode in Daniel's life when the response to his prayer was not as forthcoming. We will see that we, like Daniel, will often have to *battle* in prayer against the spiritual forces that are opposing us.

BATTLING IN PRAYER

We need to know who our adversary is, what his strategy is, and how we are to protect ourselves defensively while going on the offense against him.

Anne Graham Lotz

The savannas of Africa are filled with all kinds of dangerous animals—hyenas, warthogs, wildebeests, rhinos, and the like. But there is one predator that rises above the rest when people think of dangerous predators: the *lion*. Why is this creature so feared? Perhaps it has to do with the way lions hunt. Lions generally work in groups of three to eight. They like to silently stalk their prey, moving under the cover of the grasslands or the night. They work to isolate the weak from the pack. When they are able to do so, they move in quickly for the kill.

In the Bible, Peter refers to Satan, your enemy, as this kind of creature. He writes, "Be self-controlled and alert. Your enemy the devil prowls around like a roaring lion looking for someone to devour" (1 Peter 5:8). Like a lion, Satan works with the forces under his control to defeat you in prayer. He lurks in the shadows, studying ways to disrupt your communication with God and frustrate your efforts at doing His will. He is persistent in his attempts to isolate you from other believers to make you feel alone. His sole purpose is to devour—to discourage, discredit, and defeat you—especially in prayer.

This explains why prayer so often feels like hard work. When you enter into conversation with God, you are also entering into a *battle* against the spiritual forces of this world. Your enemy is crafty. He will try to fill your mind with distractions or create chaos to keep you off your knees. He will try to discourage you—just like he tried to do with Daniel in today's video session—and make you feel as if your prayers are ineffective. Or he will stroke your pride and self-esteem and try to convince you that you don't really need God.

Fortunately, God's Word says "the one who is in you is greater than the one who is in the world" (1 John 4:4). Satan is a formidable foe, but he is also a defeated foe. Furthermore, God has not left you defenseless in the battle. He has equipped you with spiritual armor to protect you from the enemy's attacks and a powerful weapon to repel the enemy's onslaughts. And over it all, He has given you the covering of *prayer*.

In this final Bible study, we are going to go outside Daniel's story and focus on what the apostle Paul reveals about the spiritual battle. In particular, look for descriptions of our adversary, our armor, and our assignment.

PRE-SESSION BIBLE STUDY

Begin this final week by reading Ephesians 6:10–20, and then work through each of the personal Bible studies using the steps you learned in the opening workshop. You will review the lessons and personal applications during your group session and then watch the teaching from Anne.

STUDY 1

STEP 1	STEP 2
Read God's Word	*What Does God's Word Say?*
Passage: Ephesians 6:10–11	*(List the facts.)*

10 Finally, be strong in the Lord and in his mighty power.

11 Put on the full armor of God so that you can take your stand against the devil's schemes.

STEP 3

What Does God's Word Mean?
(Learn the lessons.)

STEP 4

What Does God's Word Mean in My Life?
(Listen to His voice.)

STEP 5

How Will I Respond to God's Word?
(Live it out!)

Name: _____ Date: _____

STUDY 2

STEP 1	STEP 2
Read God's Word	*What Does God's Word Say?*
Passage: Ephesians 6:12–13	*(List the facts.)*

12 For our struggle is not against flesh and blood, but against the rulers, against the authorities, against the powers of this dark world and against the spiritual forces of evil in the heavenly realms.

13 Therefore put on the full armor of God, so that when the day of evil comes, you may be able to stand your ground, and after you have done everything, to stand.

STEP 3

What Does God's Word Mean?
(Learn the lessons.)

STEP 4

What Does God's Word Mean in My Life?
(Listen to His voice.)

STEP 5

How Will I Respond to God's Word?
(Live it out!)

Name: _____ Date: _____

STUDY 3

STEP 1	STEP 2
Read God's Word	*What Does God's Word Say?*
Passage: Ephesians 6:14–15	*(List the facts.)*

14 Stand firm then, with the belt of truth buckled around your waist, with the breastplate of righteousness in place,

15 and with your feet fitted with the readiness that comes from the gospel of peace.

STEP 3
What Does God's Word Mean?
(Learn the lessons.)

STEP 4
What Does God's Word Mean in My Life?
(Listen to His voice.)

STEP 5

How Will I Respond to God's Word?
(Live it out!)

Name: _____ Date: _____

STUDY 4

STEP 1

Read God's Word

Passage: Ephesians 6:16–17

16 In addition to all this, take up the shield of faith, with which you can extinguish all the flaming arrows of the evil one.

17 Take the helmet of salvation and the sword of the Spirit, which is the word of God.

STEP 2

What Does God's Word Say?

(List the facts.)

STEP 3
What Does God's Word Mean?
(Learn the lessons.)

STEP 4
What Does God's Word Mean in My Life?
(Listen to His voice.)

STEP 5

How Will I Respond to God's Word?
(Live it out!)

Name: _____ Date: _____

STUDY 5

STEP 1	STEP 2

STEP 1

Read God's Word

Passage: Ephesians 6:18–20

18 And pray in the Spirit on all occasions with all kinds of prayers and requests. With this in mind, be alert and always keep on praying for all the saints.

19 Pray also for me, that whenever I open my mouth, words may be given me so that I will fearlessly make known the mystery of the gospel,

20 for which I am an ambassador in chains. Pray that I may declare it fearlessly, as I should.

STEP 2

What Does God's Word Say?

(List the facts.)

STEP 3

What Does God's Word Mean?
(Learn the lessons.)

STEP 4

What Does God's Word Mean in My Life?
(Listen to His voice.)

STEP 5

How Will I Respond to God's Word?
(Live it out!)

Name: _____ Date: _____

WATCH VIDEO SESSION 6—
BATTLING IN PRAYER

Watch video streaming or on DVD.

Use this space to take notes if you like:

GROUP DISCUSSION QUESTIONS

Open your group discussion sharing something in the video teaching that was either striking or was new to you altogether.

1. How does it change your view of prayer when you see it as a spiritual battle?

2. What are some subtle things the enemy does to try to keep you from praying?

3. How does the enemy try to convince you the battle is not serious?

4. Why is it critical to wrap yourself in God's Word before confronting the enemy?

5. In what ways does the Word of God serve as your weapon in the fight?

CHOICES

This week, you studied Ephesians 6:6–20. Coupled with the video teaching on Daniel 10, we can clearly see how prayer is spiritual warfare against a crafty foe. Think back on how you responded to this passage of Scripture (step 5 in your daily studies). Write down some areas you need to work on to better view prayer as a battle and be more intentional in your time with God. Then, go back and review all the "choices" you made throughout this study. Is there anything you now want to add or delete? Is there any further insight or additional choice you want to make? If so, write those items in the blocks provided on pages 112–113.

What I will do to approach prayer as a serious battle . . .

What I will do to prevail in prayer . . .

What I will do with what I discover as I examine my heart . . .

What I will do to pray under compulsion . . .

What I will do to prepare for prayer . . .

WRAPPING UP

In Ephesians 6:12, the apostle Paul states that our struggle "is not against flesh and blood, but against the rulers, against the authorities, against the powers of this dark world and against the spiritual forces of evil in the heavenly realms." It is important for us not to underestimate our enemy, for he is crafty and looks for weaknesses in our armor to exploit. But neither should we fall into despair, for we know that we serve the One who has ultimately defeated our enemy.

> *[Jesus] warned His followers that, "In this world you will have trouble. But take heart! I have overcome the world" (John 16:33). And because He has overcome, you and I will overcome also. At the end of human history as we know it, when the world melts down and seems totally dominated and ruled by the devil himself, the followers of Jesus will overcome the enemy "by the blood of the Lamb and by the word of their testimony" (Revelation 12:11).*

—Anne Graham Lotz, *The Daniel Prayer*, page 258

As you pray the Daniel Prayer in the weeks and months ahead, remember that you are at war! So, when you run into those times when you find it difficult to keep your commitment to pray, it's important not to quit. When you find your mind wandering and you struggle to keep focused in prayer, it's critical not to give up.

When your prayers seem weak and ineffective, it's vital to stay the course. For as Daniel's story reveals, your prayers can move Heaven!

As we conclude this study, consider your need to battle in prayer. What are some obstacles the enemy has placed in your path that you need to overcome? What are some barriers that need to be removed so you can move forward? On the lines below, write out your own heart-prayer to God. Ask the God of Daniel for His intervention as you seek to follow His will, and receive the answers to prayer He has already chosen to give you. Heaven will be moved! And I pray, your world and our nation will be changed! For the glory of His Name!

MY PRAYER

SIMPLIFIED AND ABBREVIATED BIBLE STUDY

As mentioned at the beginning of the guide, there is an alternate "track" that you and your group can follow if your meeting time is more limited (forty-five minutes in length). For this track, you will study only a few key verses with your group each session, and no homework assignments will be required.

> *Note: The session 1 Bible Study Workshop will be the same regardless of which track you and your group take.*

PREPARING FOR PRAYER

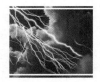

Just as an athlete can't expect to win by showing up at game time without having practiced, the commitment to pray doesn't just happen. It requires preparation.

Anne Graham Lotz

BIBLE STUDY

Begin this session by having someone in the group read Daniel 6:10 aloud (see next page), and then work through each of the steps together following the method you learned in the workshop. Once you have spent a few minutes discussing the passage, watch the teaching from Anne.

STEP 1

Read God's Word

Passage: Daniel 6:10

10 Now when Daniel learned that the decree had been published, he went home to his upstairs room where the windows opened toward Jerusalem. Three times a day he got down on his knees and prayed, giving thanks to his God, just as he had done before.

STEP 2

What Does God's Word Say?

(List the facts.)

STEP 3

What Does God's Word Mean?
(Learn the lessons.)

STEP 4

What Does God's Word Mean in My Life?
(Listen to His voice.)

STEP 5

How Will I Respond to God's Word?
(Live it out!)

Name: _____ Date: _____

WATCH VIDEO SESSION 2—
PREPARING FOR PRAYER

Watch video streaming or on DVD.

Use this space to take notes if you like:

GROUP DISCUSSION QUESTIONS

Open your group discussion sharing something in the video teaching that was either striking or was new to you altogether.

1. What encouraged or challenged you in this study?

2. What did you learn that was a new thought to you?

WRAPPING UP

Three times a day, when Daniel went to his designated place for prayer, he opened his windows toward Jerusalem. The poignant gesture revealed not only the longing in his heart for his city and his people, but also his exclusive focus on the God of Abraham, Isaac, and Jacob. The God of his fathers. The God who had been with him throughout his lifetime, for over eighty years. The one, true, living God whom Daniel worshiped and served and obeyed.

—Anne Graham Lotz, *The Daniel Prayer*, page 38

Daniel had cultivated a lifetime habit of prayer and was unwilling to compromise even the smallest detail in his worship to the Lord. Even though he was in captivity and under constant threat, three times a day—without fail—he expressed his thankfulness to God. Today, as you prepare to move forward, consider what it would look like for you to cultivate such an attitude toward God and during the week write out a prayer in response.

MOVING FORWARD

Once you take the first step of preparing a time, place, atmosphere, and attitude for prayer, you are ready for the next step. You must now consider what *prompts* you to pray the kind of heartfelt cry to God that Daniel prayed for others. We will examine this aspect of the Daniel Prayer in the next session.

PROMPTING IN PRAYER

The Daniel Prayer is not just venting to God. . . . It is an outpouring of heartfelt emotion and passionate pleading based on God's Word as we hold Him to His promises.

Anne Graham Lotz

BIBLE STUDY

Begin this session by having someone in the group read Daniel 9:2–3 aloud (see next page), and then work through each of the steps together following the method you learned in the workshop. Once you have spent a few minutes discussing the passage, watch the teaching from Anne.

STEP 1

Read God's Word

Passage: Daniel 9:2–3

2 in the first year of his reign, I, Daniel, understood from the Scriptures, according to the word of the LORD given to Jeremiah the prophet, that the desolation of Jerusalem would last seventy years.

3 So I turned to the Lord God and pleaded with him in prayer and petition, in fasting, and in sackcloth and ashes.

STEP 2

What Does God's Word Say?

(List the facts.)

STEP 3

What Does God's Word Mean?
(Learn the lessons.)

STEP 4

What Does God's Word Mean in My Life?
(Listen to His voice.)

STEP 5

How Will I Respond to God's Word?
(Live it out!)

Name: _____ Date: _____

WATCH VIDEO SESSION 3—
PROMPTING IN PRAYER

Watch video streaming or on DVD.

Use this space to take notes if you like:

GROUP DISCUSSION QUESTIONS

Open your group discussion sharing something in the video teaching that was either striking or was new to you altogether.

1. What encouraged or challenged you in this study?

2. What did you learn that was a new thought to you?

WRAPPING UP

[God] is the Center-point. When our prayers are focused, regardless of what life throws at us, whether it's a long, hard climb to the top of our profession or career, or the steady trail of perseverance as we set out to achieve our goals, or the confusion and lost feeling that can envelop us when we find ourselves in a thicket of problems and pressures and pain—if our prayers are focused on the living God, they will make a difference.

—Anne Graham Lotz, *The Daniel Prayer*, page 65

Daniel had this type of laser-focus when he responded to the promptings he felt to pray for God's people. Before he spoke even a word, he "turned to the Lord God" (Daniel 9:3). The Lord was his Center-point, and regardless of the situation, he knew that God would deliver on His promises. Today, consider what would prompt you to pray as Daniel prayed. What would it look like for you to center on God privately, sincerely, desperately, and humbly? What promises from the Bible do you need God to bring to mind? During the upcoming week, write out a prayer to God in response.

MOVING FORWARD

Once you consider what compels you to pray and how you should be centered on God when you pray, you are ready for the next step. You should now consider what it looks like to *plead* in prayer as Daniel did for his people. We will examine this aspect of the Daniel Prayer in the next session.

PLEADING
IN PRAYER

*Daniel was confident of who God was.
He knew God belonged to him and that he
belonged to God. This covenant relationship with
God was the bedrock of the Daniel Prayer.*

Anne Graham Lotz

BIBLE STUDY

Begin this session by having someone in the group read Daniel 9:4–5 aloud (see next page), and then work through each of the steps together following the method you learned in the workshop. Once you have spent a few minutes discussing the passage, watch the teaching from Anne.

STEP 1

Read God's Word

Passage: Daniel 9:4–5

⁴ I prayed to the LORD my God and confessed: "O Lord, the great and awesome God, who keeps his covenant of love with all who love him and obey his commands,

⁵ "we have sinned and done wrong. We have been wicked and have rebelled; we have turned away from your commands and laws."

STEP 2

What Does God's Word Say?

(List the facts.)

STEP 3

What Does God's Word Mean?
(Learn the lessons.)

STEP 4

What Does God's Word Mean in My Life?
(Listen to His voice.)

STEP 5

How Will I Respond to God's Word?
(Live it out!)

Name: _____ Date: _____

WATCH VIDEO SESSION 4—
PLEADING IN PRAYER

Watch video streaming or on DVD.

Use this space to take notes if you like:

GROUP DISCUSSION QUESTIONS

Open your group discussion sharing something in the video teaching that was either striking or was new to you altogether.

1. What encouraged or challenged you in this study?

2. What did you learn that was a new thought to you?

WRAPPING UP

I think one reason some of us, myself included, don't examine our hearts for sin is because we are so afraid we will find it. One thing I have discovered is that it takes courage to look deep within to see what God sees. It's painful to acknowledge that we're not as good, righteous, pure, or holy as we thought.

—Anne Graham Lotz, *The Daniel Prayer*, pages 129–130

Before you apply the Daniel Prayer to the sins of others, it is important to take a moment to look at the sins in your own life. Would you be courageous enough, after reading three times through the list of sins included in the back of this study guide, to confess your sin in a heart-prayer to God expressing your sorrow and asking for His forgiveness? During the upcoming week, write out that prayer to God.

MOVING FORWARD

Once you have examined your understanding of God and your relationship with Him, and have confessed your own sins with clarity, you are ready for the next step. You will now consider what is required to *prevail* in prayer until you receive an answer from God. We will examine this aspect of the Daniel Prayer in the next session.

SESSION 5
SIMPLIFIED STUDY

PREVAILING IN PRAYER

Drive the stake of your faith deep down into God's promises. Don't quit. Don't give up. Don't give in. Don't collapse. Don't settle for less than prayer that moves Heaven and changes nations.

Anne Graham Lotz

BIBLE STUDY

Begin this session by having someone in the group read Daniel 9:21–23 aloud (see next page), and then work through each of the steps together following the method you learned in the workshop. Once you have spent a few minutes discussing the passage, watch the teaching from Anne.

STEP 1

Read God's Word
Passage: Daniel 9:21–23

21 While I was still in prayer, Gabriel, the man I had seen in the earlier vision, came to me in swift flight about the time of the evening sacrifice.

22 He instructed me and said to me, "Daniel, I have now come to give you insight and understanding.

23 "As soon as you began to pray, an answer was given, which I have come to tell you, for you are highly esteemed. Therefore, consider the message and understand the vision . . ."

STEP 2

What Does God's Word Say?
(List the facts.)

STEP 3
What Does God's Word Mean?
(Learn the lessons.)

STEP 4
What Does God's Word Mean in My Life?
(Listen to His voice.)

STEP 5

How Will I Respond to God's Word?
(Live it out!)

Name: _____ Date: _____

WATCH VIDEO SESSION 5—
PREVAILING IN PRAYER

Watch video streaming or on DVD.

Use this space to take notes if you like:

GROUP DISCUSSION QUESTIONS

Open your group discussion sharing something in the video teaching that was either striking or was new to you altogether.

1. What encouraged or challenged you in this study?

2. What did you learn that was a new thought to you?

WRAPPING UP

To prevail in prayer . . . [is] to put your arms of faith about your Father's neck and cling tightly to Him until He blesses you. But to prevail, you must be sure that what you are praying for is something you know God wants to give you. And how do you know what He wants to give you? You base your prayer on God's Word. Then you hold Him to it through prevailing prayer.

—Anne Graham Lotz, *The Daniel Prayer*, page 172

Remember that when Daniel made his request to God, he was praying back a promise the Lord had already made in the Scriptures. Daniel could approach God confidently because he knew that he was praying for something that God already wanted to give. His act of prevailing in prayer was a means by which he was holding God accountable to His Word. Today, consider what it would look like for you to pray in the same way. Then pray accordingly. In the upcoming week, write a prayer to God based on the promises you have discovered in God's Word.

MOVING FORWARD

When you pray the Daniel Prayer, you may receive an immediate answer to your request. However, there will be times when prevailing in prayer doesn't lead to an instantaneous response. In the final session of this study, we will examine another episode in Daniel's life when the response to his prayer was not as forthcoming. We will see that we, like Daniel, will often have to *battle* in prayer against the spiritual forces that are opposing us.

BATTLING IN PRAYER

We need to know who our adversary is, what his strategy is, and how we are to protect ourselves defensively while going on the offense against him.

Anne Graham Lotz

BIBLE STUDY

Begin this session by having someone in the group read Daniel 10:12–13 aloud (see next page), and then work through each of the steps together following the method you learned in the workshop. Once you have spent a few minutes discussing the passage, watch the teaching from Anne.

STEP 1

Read God's Word

Passage: Daniel 10:12–13

12 Then he continued, "Do not be afraid, Daniel. Since the first day that you set your mind to gain understanding and to humble yourself before your God, your words were heard, and I have come in response to them.

13 "But the prince of the Persian kingdom resisted me twenty-one days. Then Michael, one of the chief princes, came to help me, because I was detained there with the king of Persia."

STEP 2

What Does God's Word Say?

(List the facts.)

STEP 3

What Does God's Word Mean?
(Learn the lessons.)

STEP 4

What Does God's Word Mean in My Life?
(Listen to His voice.)

STEP 5

How Will I Respond to God's Word?
(Live it out!)

Name: _____ Date: _____

WATCH VIDEO SESSION 6—
BATTLING IN PRAYER

Watch video streaming or on DVD.

Use this space to take notes if you like:

GROUP DISCUSSION QUESTIONS

Open your group discussion sharing something in the video teaching that was either striking or was new to you altogether.

1. What encouraged or challenged you in this study?

2. What did you learn that was a new thought to you?

WRAPPING UP

In Ephesians 6:12, the apostle Paul states that our struggle "is not against flesh and blood, but against the rulers, against the authorities, against the powers of this dark world and against the spiritual forces of evil in the heavenly realms." It is important for us not to underestimate our enemy, for he is crafty and looks for weaknesses in our armor to exploit. But neither should we fall into despair, for we know that we serve the One who has ultimately defeated our enemy.

> *[Jesus] warned His followers that, "In this world you will have trouble. But take heart! I have overcome the world" (John 16:33). And because He has overcome, you and I will overcome also. At the end of human history as we know it, when the world melts down and seems totally dominated and ruled by the devil himself, the followers of Jesus will overcome the enemy "by the blood of the Lamb and by the word of their testimony" (Revelation 12:11).*

> —Anne Graham Lotz, *The Daniel Prayer*, page 258

As you pray the Daniel Prayer in the weeks and months ahead, remember that you are at war! So, when you run into those times when you find it difficult to keep your commitment to pray, it's important not to quit. When you find your mind wandering and you struggle to keep focused in prayer, it's critical not to give up. When your prayers seem weak and ineffective, it's vital to stay the course. For as Daniel's story reveals, your prayers can move Heaven!

As you conclude this study, consider your need to battle in prayer. What are some obstacles the enemy has placed in your path that you need to overcome? What are some barriers that need to be removed so you can move forward? Ask the God of Daniel for His intervention as you seek to follow His will, and receive the answers to prayer He has already chosen to give you. Heaven will be moved, and your world and our nation will be changed! For the glory of His Name!

LIST OF SINS

Ingratitude. Failure to thank God for the favors He has bestowed both before and after salvation. What blessings or answered prayer have you neglected to thank God for?

Losing Your Love for God. Loving people or things more than you love God. Have you lost your first love for Jesus?

Neglect of Bible Reading. Pushing daily Bible reading aside due to an over-full schedule or being preoccupied with other things as you read. How long has it been since reading your Bible was a delight? Do you remember what it says when you are finished?

Unbelief. Refusing to believe that God will give you what He has promised (which is the same as accusing Him of lying). What promise do you think He will not keep?

Neglect of Prayer. Offering prayer up to God as spiritual chatter, fantasy, wishful thinking, or daydreaming. Do you offer prayers without fervent, focused faith?

Lack of Concern for the Salvation of Others. Standing by and watching people on their way to hell without caring enough to warn them, pray for them, or admit that is where they are going. Have you become so politically correct that you don't apply the gospel to those you know and love? Do you think it is someone else's responsibility to tell them?

Neglect of Family. Putting yourself and your needs before those of your loved ones. What effort are you making, and what habits have you established, for your family's spiritual good when it requires personal sacrifice?

Love of the World and Material Things. Thinking of your possessions as your own instead of blessings and gifts from God. Do you believe your money is yours and that you can spend it as you choose without asking God?

Pride. Over-concern about outward appearances and thinking you are better than someone else. Are you offended, or even irritated, if others don't notice certain things about you? How do you react when people say you are wrong?

Envy. Jealousy of those who seem more fruitful, gifted, or recognizable than you. Do you struggle with hearing somebody else praised?

A Critical Spirit. Speaking about others in a manner that is empty of grace and love. Do you find fault with others? Do you set standards for them?

Slander. Telling the truth about a person with the intention of causing people to think less of him or her. Whose faults, real or imagined, about others have you discussed behind their backs?

Lack of Seriousness toward God. Not showing God the honor and respect He is due. Do you show disrespect for God by sleeping through your prayer time or showing up late for church as though He doesn't matter? Do you give God the left-overs of your emotions, time, thoughts, or money?

Lying. Saying anything that is contrary to the unvarnished truth. What have you said to impress someone that wasn't the whole truth or was an exaggeration of the truth?

Cheating. Treating others in a way you wouldn't want to be treated. Have you stopped short of treating others the way you would want to be treated?

Hypocrisy. Pretending to be something you are not. Are you pretending to be anything you are not?

Robbing God. Wasting time on things that have no eternal value or exercising your God-given gifts and talents for a fee. What are you *not* doing for God that you are willing to do for others—for a price?

Temper. Losing patience with a child, coworker, friend, spouse, staff member, or anyone else. What cross words have you spoken lately?

Bad temper. Losing control of your emotions, thoughts, and words so that you abuse someone else verbally. Have you lost your temper recently?

Hindering Others. Taking other people's time needlessly or destroying their confidence because you hold them to an unreasonably high standard. Have you done this?

Arrogance. Accepting God's forgiveness while refusing to forgive yourself or somebody else. Have you been guilty of this lately?

THE
DANIEL
PRAYER

PRAYER THAT MOVES HEAVEN
AND CHANGES NATIONS

FACILITATOR'S GUIDE

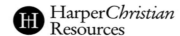

Harper*Christian*
Resources

CONTENTS

THANK YOU

Thank you for serving as the facilitator for the participants who will join you in this study. While I will have the privilege of speaking to them through the video series, your leadership is essential. Your thoughtful and loving guidance will encourage them to consistently do their Bible study during the week and feel comfortable sharing their discoveries in your group. Please be assured that I, and others on this curriculum development team, have been praying for you.

> I thank my God every time I remember you. In all my prayers for all of you, I always pray with joy because of your partnership in the gospel from the first day until now, being confident of this, that he who began a good work in you will carry it on to completion until the day of Christ Jesus. (Philippians 1:3–6)

As you lead others to develop a more effective prayer life, I pray that you will experience the fullness of God's blessing and that you, too, will discover how to pray in a manner that moves Heaven and changes nations.

For His Glory,

FOR STARTERS

Please take a few minutes to read this helpful information before you begin *The Daniel Prayer* study. It should answer most of the questions you may have.

HOW TO ACCESS THE VIDEOS

- There is a **DVD available for purchase** in addition to the study guide, if DVD is your preferred method of watching the video teaching. **Streaming video** access is included with this study guide. There is a streaming video access code and instructions on how to access all of the video sessions on the inside front cover of this study guide.

- Simply go to studygateway.com/redeem to set up your account and enter your access code to add this study to your new Bible study library.

- Each time you wish to view a video, simply log in to studygateway.com/login and click on the session or study you wish to view.

- All of your HarperChristian Resources Bible studies with streaming access will be added to your library as you do more studies and redeem the appropriate codes.

WHAT OTHER MATERIALS ARE NEEDED?

The following materials will be needed for a successful small group time:

- A computer with monitor or a television with a DVD player

- A watch, clock, or cellphone with alarm (to monitor the time)

- *The Daniel Prayer Study Guide* (one per group member) with streaming video access. (DVD available separately if preferred.)

- A Bible (one per group member)

- Pens or pencils (enough for everyone)

- Optional: *The Daniel Prayer* book by Anne Graham Lotz (recommended for leaders, but optional for participants)

WHAT ARE THE TWO TRACKS FOR THIS STUDY?

There are two approaches you can use for the weekly meetings based on your group dynamics:

- **Main Study:** For the main track, the group members will study five days' worth of Bible study readings using the approach outlined in the Bible Study Workshop. You will then lead them in a discussion of portions of these passages, watch the video, go through the more extensive discussion questions, and close with a Choices activity that the members will do together. This track is ideal for more comprehensive group studies with extended meeting times.

- **Simplified and Abbreviated Study:** For the alternate track, the group members will study only a few key verses in their group each session, and no homework assignments will be required. You will then lead them in a discussion of these passages, watch the video, and go through the condensed discussion questions. This track is ideal for groups with more limited meeting time, such as a workplace lunchtime setting.

  Note: The session 1 Bible Study Workshop demonstrates the Bible study method to be used for both options.

GOOD TO KNOW

Here are a few additional items to keep in mind as you lead your group:

- **Your Role as Facilitator:** As the facilitator, your role is to take care of your guests by managing the behind-the-scenes details so that when everyone arrives, they can just enjoy their time together. Your role is *not* to answer all the questions or reteach the content—the video and study guide will do much of the work. You want to guide the group and make it a place where people can process, question, and reflect on the Bible readings and the teachings.

- **Setting and Time:** This study can work equally well in church or home groups. The first session is planned to be 90 minutes in length, while the subsequent sessions are approximately 60 minutes (or 45 minutes for the alternate track). In more formal, time-sensitive church settings, you will likely need to follow the time frames provided in the session outline more closely in order to finish all the content. In less formal home settings, you can "round off" time frames and still end up with about an hour of study material. In either case, remember these are suggested time frames and are open to adjustment as you see fit.

- **Hospitality:** Regardless of where you conduct the study, create an environment that is conducive to sharing and learning. Make sure there is enough comfortable seating for everyone and, if possible, arrange the seats in a semicircle so everyone can see the video. This will make the transition between the video and group conversation more natural. Consider offering simple refreshments to create a welcoming atmosphere, and make sure your media technology is working properly before the session begins.

WEEKLY PREPARATION

As the facilitator, there are a few things you many want to do to prepare for each meeting:

- **Read through the lesson:** This will help you to become familiar with the content and know how to structure the discussion times.

- **Decide which questions you want to discuss:** Depending on the track you follow and how you structure your group time, you may not be able to cover every question in the group discussion section. Select the questions ahead of time that you absolutely want the group to discuss in depth.

- **Be familiar with the questions you want to discuss:** When the group meets you will be watching the clock, so make sure you are familiar with the study questions you have selected.

- **Pray for your group:** Pray for your group members by name throughout the week and ask God to lead them as they study His Word.

- **Bring extra supplies to your meeting:** The group members should bring their own pens for writing notes, but it's a good idea to have extras available for those who forget. You may also want to bring additional paper and Bibles.

GROUP DYNAMICS

Leading a group is highly rewarding, but that doesn't mean you will not encounter any challenges along the way. Discussions can get off track. Group members may not be sensitive to the ideas of others. Some may express comments that result in disagreements. To help ease this strain on you and the group, consider the following ground rules:

- **Off topic:** When someone raises a question or comment that is off the main topic, suggest you deal with it another time, or, if you feel led to go in that direction, let the group know you will be spending some time discussing it.

- **Don't know the answer:** If someone asks a question you don't know how to answer, admit it and move on. At your discretion, feel free to invite group members to comment on questions that call for personal experience.

- **Dominating discussion:** If you find one or two people are dominating the discussion time, direct questions to others in the group. Outside the group time, ask the more dominating members to help you draw out the quieter ones. Work to make them a part of the solution instead of the problem.

- **Disagreements:** When a disagreement occurs, encourage group members to process the matter in love. Have those on opposite sides restate what they heard the other side say about the matter, and then invite each side to evaluate if that perception is accurate. It's most important that the answers given are based on the passages of Scripture studied.

When these situations arise, guide your group to follow the words from the Bible: "Love one another" (John 13:34), "As far as it depends on you, live at peace with everyone" (Romans 12:18), and "Be quick to listen, slow to speak and slow to become angry" (James 1:19).

SESSION 1

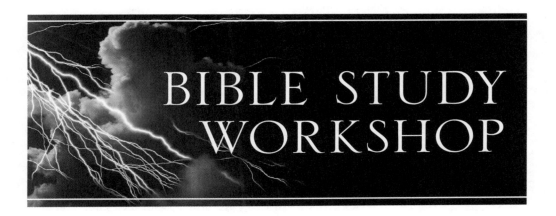

For the best experience in facilitating this study, it's important to preview the video for session 1 and complete all the written exercises in this study guide prior to leading your group. Familiarize yourself with the session outline and gather the necessary materials. Pray for the participants by name (if known). Pray Ephesians 1:17–18 for them, that God will open their hearts to His Word, and they will get to know Him better as a result of the Spirit's revelation.

SESSION OUTLINE (90 MINUTES)

I. Introduction/Opening Prayer (5 minutes)

II. Explanation of Bible Study Sessions (3 minutes)

III. Video Teaching and Group Work (77 minutes)

    A. Opening and Teaching on Steps 1–2 (14 minutes)

    B. Group Work on Steps 1–2 (8 minutes)

    C. Review of Steps 1–2 and Teaching on Step 3 (2 minutes)

    D. Group Work on Step 3 (15 minutes)

E. Review of Step 3 and Teaching on Step 4 (13 minutes)

F. Group Work on Step 4 (5 minutes)

G. Review of Step 4 and Teaching on Step 5 (12 minutes)

H. Group Work on Step 5 (2 minutes)

I. Review of Step 5 and Closing (6 minutes)

IV. Wrapping Up and Next Steps (5 minutes)

INTRODUCTION/OPENING PRAYER (5 MINUTES)

Take a few moments as this opening session begins to introduce yourself to anyone in the group you do not know and give your contact information. If it can be done quickly, ask the participants to introduce themselves. It may be helpful in a larger group to provide nametags. To save time, you can have the nametags pre-printed with their names on one side, and your name and contact information on the other side. Ensure the participants have a copy of the study guide. Pray that God would use the coming hour to help everyone present to become more effective students and doers of His Word.

EXPLANATION OF BIBLE STUDY SESSIONS (3 MINUTES)

Explain that this first session in *The Daniel Prayer* is unique, as Anne will describe a method for studying the Bible that the participants will use during their personal quiet time throughout the study. Ask them to turn to page 20 in their study guide and follow along. (Note: If you are following the alternate track, it will serve as the basis for discussion.) During this opening session, which will be approximately 90 minutes in length, the group members will watch the video and complete the work found on pages 22–23.

VIDEO TEACHING AND GROUP WORK (77 MINUTES)

Show the video, following the instructions given by Anne during the session. Note that you will be stopping the video periodically for the participants to complete each of the steps.

WRAPPING UP AND NEXT STEPS (5 MINUTES)

Tell the group members that next week they will begin to explore the Daniel Prayer by studying what is needed to prepare for prayer. If you are following the main track, refer group members to the Pre-Session Bible Study found on pages 28–37, which describes the Bible study assignment for session 2, and ask them to complete the studies before the next session. (If you are following the alternate track, refer the group members to pages 118–119 and ask them to read the passage before the next session.) Close your time in prayer.

MAIN BIBLE STUDY TRACK

For the main track, your group members will study five days' worth of selected Scripture readings in their study guides between the weekly meetings. At the start of each session, you will lead a short review of the facts, lessons, and most meaningful questions they drew from the passage they studied. You will then play the video (with the group members taking notes), discuss the questions listed for this track, and lead a short "Choices" activity. To use this track, your meeting time must be a least **60 minutes** in order to cover all the necessary material.

> *Note:* For this track, passages outside of Daniel are used. They have been selected because they underscore the theme for that week's particular study:

SESSION 2: PREPARING FOR PRAYER . . . . MATTHEW 6:5–18

SESSION 3: PROMPTING IN PRAYER. . . . . 2 CHRONICLES 6:40–7:22

SESSION 4: PLEADING IN PRAYER . . . . NEHEMIAH 1:1–2:9

SESSION 5: PREVAILING IN PRAYER. . . . . .2 CHRONICLES 20:1–30

SESSION 6: BATTLING IN PRAYER . . . . EPHESIANS 6:10–20

SESSION 2

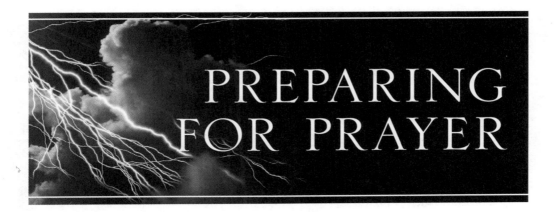

PREPARING FOR PRAYER

Preview the video for session 2 before your meeting and complete all the written exercises in the study guide. If possible, read the introduction and chapter 1 of *The Daniel Prayer* for more background information on the teaching covered during the session. Familiarize yourself with the session outline and gather the necessary materials. Remember also to pray for the participants who will be attending, asking God to help them as they go through the steps on preparing for prayer.

SESSION OUTLINE (60 MINUTES)

I. Review of Pre-Session Bible Study (15 minutes)

   A. Study 1: Matthew 6:5

   B. Study 2: Matthew 6:6

   C. Study 3: Matthew 6:7–8

   D. Study 4: Matthew 6:9–13

   E. Study 5: Matthew 6:14–18

II. Video Teaching (18 minutes)

   A. A prepared place to pray . . .

   B. A prepared time to pray . . .

   C. A prepared atmosphere for prayer . . .

   D. A prepared attitude for prayer . . .

III. Group Discussion (17 minutes)

   A. What is the "Daniel Prayer"? How is it different from other kinds of prayer?

   B. What is the best place for you to meet God each day in prayer?

   C. What is the best time for you to set aside for prayer?

   D. How can you create an atmosphere that is more conducive for prayer?

   E. What are some ways you can cultivate an attitude of gratitude when you come to God in prayer?

IV. Choices Activity (5 minutes)

V. Wrapping Up and Moving Forward (5 minutes)

REVIEW OF PRE-SESSION BIBLE STUDY (15 MINUTES)

Welcome any new participants, and then refer the group to their notes on pages 28–37. As time allows, have one member share the **facts** he or she drew from each verse (Step 2). Then have several different members share the following:

- The **lessons** they learned from each verse (Step 3).

- The most meaningful **question** they wrote out in response to Step 4, citing the verse on which the question was based.

- Their outstanding **takeaway** in Step 5.

VIDEO TEACHING (18 MINUTES)

Watch the teaching video for session 2. Refer the group members to the outline on page 38 and remind them there is space to take notes.

GROUP DISCUSSION (17 MINUTES)

Refer to the Group Discussion questions on pages 38–39 to stimulate discussion on the topics presented during the video teaching. Ask the group members to share any personal encouragement, challenge, or inspiration they received as they watched.

CHOICES ACTIVITY (5 MINUTES)

Ask group members to think back on how they responded to the passage of Scripture they studied this week. Encourage them to take a few minutes to complete the Choices activity found on page 39 as a way of making sure they are not just "hearers" but "doers" of the Word.

WRAPPING UP AND MOVING FORWARD (5 MINUTES)

Conclude by asking the group members to write out their prayers to God on page 41, expressing their gratitude to the Lord in spite of the challenges or trials they are facing. Refer them to the Pre-Session Bible Study found on pages 46–55, which describes the Bible study assignment for session 3. Remind them to read the passage and complete the studies before the next session. Close in prayer.

SESSION 3

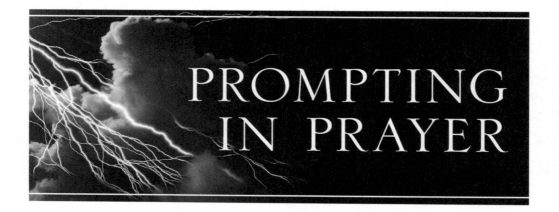

PROMPTING IN PRAYER

Preview the video for session 3 before your meeting and complete all the written exercises in the study guide. If possible, read chapters 2 and 3 of *The Daniel Prayer* for more background information on the teaching covered during the session. Familiarize yourself with the session outline and gather the necessary materials. Remember also to pray for the participants who will be attending, asking God to help them as they go through the steps on being prompted to pray the Daniel Prayer.

SESSION OUTLINE (60 MINUTES)

I. Review of Pre-Session Bible Study (13 minutes)

    A. Study 1: 2 Chronicles 6:40–42

    B. Study 2: 2 Chronicles 7:1–6

    C. Study 3: 2 Chronicles 7:7–10

    D. Study 4: 2 Chronicles 7:11–16

    E. Study 5: 2 Chronicles 7:17–22

II. Video Teaching (22 minutes)

    A. Compelled by . . .
       1. Problems in the world
       2. Promises in God's Word

    B. Centered on God . . .
       1. Privately
       2. Sincerely
       3. Desperately
       4. Humbly

III. Group Discussion (15 minutes)

    A. What situations in your life or in the world have motivated you to pray?
    B. What are some promises God has given to you in His Word that you have claimed relating to the above situation?
    C. What does it mean to "hold God to His Word" in prayer?
    D. What helps you to stay centered on God when you pray?
    E. How does humility play a part in praying the Daniel Prayer?

IV. Choices Activity (5 minutes)

V. Wrapping Up and Moving Forward (5 minutes)

REVIEW OF PRE-SESSION BIBLE STUDY (13 MINUTES)

Welcome any new participants, and then refer the group to their notes on pages 46–55. As time allows, have one member share the **facts** he or she drew from each verse (Step 2). Then have several different members share the following:

• The **lessons** they learned from each verse (Step 3).

• The most meaningful **question** they wrote out in response to Step 4, citing the verse on which the question was based.

• Their outstanding **takeaway** in Step 5.

VIDEO TEACHING (22 MINUTES)

Watch the teaching video for session 3. Refer the group members to the outline on page 56 and remind them there is space to take notes.

GROUP DISCUSSION (15 MINUTES)

Refer to the Group Discussion questions on page 57 to stimulate discussion on the topics presented during the video teaching. Ask the group members to share any personal encouragement, challenge, or inspiration they received as they watched.

CHOICES ACTIVITY (5 MINUTES)

Ask group members to think back on how they responded to the passage of Scripture they studied this week. Encourage them to take a few minutes to complete the Choices activity found on pages 57–58 as a way of making sure they are not just "hearers" but "doers" of the Word.

WRAPPING UP AND MOVING FORWARD (5 MINUTES)

Conclude by asking the group members to write out their prayers to God on page 59, focusing on the promises from the Bible that they need to pray back to the Lord. Refer them to the Pre-Session Bible Study found on pages 64–73, which describes the Bible study assignment for session 4. Remind them to read the passage and complete the studies before the next session. Close in prayer.

SESSION 4

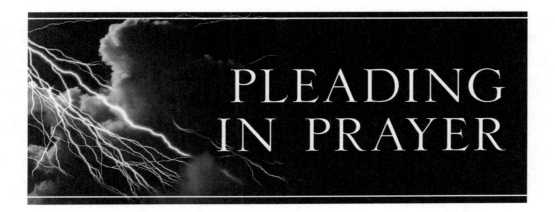

PLEADING IN PRAYER

Preview the video for session 4 before your meeting and complete all the written exercises in the study guide. If possible, read chapters 4–6 of *The Daniel Prayer* for more background information on the teaching covered during the session. Familiarize yourself with the session outline and gather the necessary materials. Remember also to pray for the participants who will be attending, asking God to help them as they go through the steps on pleading in prayer.

SESSION OUTLINE

I. Review of Pre-Session Bible Study (13 minutes)

    A. Study 1: Nehemiah 1:1–3

    B. Study 2: Nehemiah 1:4–11

    C. Study 3: Nehemiah 2:1–3

    D. Study 4: Nehemiah 2:4–6

    E. Study 5: Nehemiah 2:7–9

II. Video Teaching (25 minutes)

    A. Pleading with confidence based on your covenant relationship with God . . .

    B. Pleading with confidence based on God's character . . .

       1. God's faithfulness

       2. God's righteousness

       3. God's goodness

       4. God's greatness

    C. Pleading with contrition . . .

    D. Pleading with clarity . . .

III. Group Discussion (13 minutes)

    A. What are some of the ways you can build your confidence in God?

    B. When was a time God demonstrated His faithfulness and/or His goodness to you?

    C. When was a time God demonstrated His righteousness and/or His greatness to you?

    D. What is your reaction to the "list of sins" mentioned in the video?

    E. What are you asking God for?

IV. Choices Activity (5 minutes)

V. Wrapping Up and Moving Forward (4 minutes)

REVIEW OF PRE-SESSION BIBLE STUDY (13 MINUTES)

Refer the group to their notes on pages 64–73. As time allows, have one member share the **facts** he or she drew from each verse (Step 2). Then have several different members share the following:

• The **lessons** they learned from each verse (Step 3).

• The most meaningful **question** they wrote out in response to Step 4, citing the verse on which the question was based.

• Their outstanding **takeaway** in Step 5.

VIDEO TEACHING (25 MINUTES)

Watch the teaching video for session 4. Refer the group members to the outline on page 74 and remind them there is space to take notes.

GROUP DISCUSSION (13 MINUTES)

Refer to the Group Discussion questions on page 75 to stimulate discussion on the topics presented during the video teaching. Also ask group members to review the "List of Sins" mentioned by Anne during the teaching (pages 147–149). Ask them to share any personal encouragement, challenge, or inspiration they received as they watched the video.

CHOICES ACTIVITY (5 MINUTES)

Ask group members to think back on how they responded to the passage of Scripture they studied this week. Encourage them to take a few minutes to complete the Choices activity found on pages 75–76 as a way of making sure they are not just "hearers" but "doers" of the Word.

WRAPPING UP AND MOVING FORWARD (4 MINUTES)

Conclude by asking the group members to write out their prayers to God on page 77, focusing on what they need to do to plead in prayer. Refer them to the Pre-Session Bible Study found on pages 82–91, which describes the Bible study assignment for session 5. Remind them to read the passage and complete the studies before the next session. Close in prayer.

SESSION 5

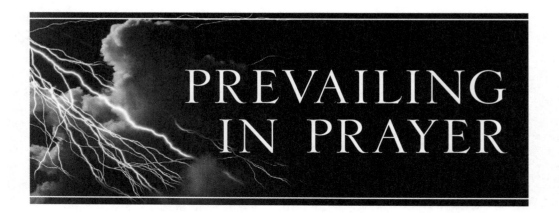

Preview the video for session 5 before your meeting and complete all the written exercises in the study guide. If possible, read chapters 7–9 of *The Daniel Prayer* for more background information on the teaching covered during the session. Familiarize yourself with the session outline and gather the necessary materials. Remember also to pray for the participants who will be attending, asking God to help them as they go through steps on prevailing in prayer.

SESSION OUTLINE

I. Review of Pre-Session Bible Study (15 minutes)

    A. Study 1: 2 Chronicles 20:1–4

    B. Study 2: 2 Chronicles 20:5–12

    C. Study 3: 2 Chronicles 20:13–19

    D. Study 4: 2 Chronicles 20:20–23

    E. Study 5: 2 Chronicles 20:24–30

II. Video Teaching (18 minutes)

    A. God answers prayer immediately . . .

    B. God answers prayer ultimately . . .

    C. God answers prayer specifically . . .

III. Group Discussion (17 minutes)

    A. What does it mean to you personally to prevail in prayer?

    B. What are some ways that you have seen God answer your prayers immediately?

    C. How has God answered your prayer ultimately? How long did you seek God in prayer before the answer came to you?

    D. In what situations have you seen God answer prayer specifically?

    E. What helps you not to be discouraged and give up when prevailing in prayer?

IV. Choices Activity (5 minutes)

V. Wrapping Up and Next Steps (5 minutes)

REVIEW OF PRE-SESSION BIBLE STUDY (15 MINUTES)

Refer the group to their notes on pages 82–91. As time allows, have one member share the **facts** he or she drew from each verse (Step 2). Then have several different members share the following:

- The **lessons** they learned from each verse (Step 3).

- The most meaningful **question** they wrote out in response to Step 4, citing the verse on which the question was based.

- Their outstanding **takeaway** in Step 5.

VIDEO TEACHING (18 MINUTES)

Watch the teaching video for session 5. Refer the group members to the outline on page 92 and remind them there is space to take notes.

GROUP DISCUSSION (17 MINUTES)

Refer to the Group Discussion questions on pages 92–93 to stimulate discussion on the topics presented during the video teaching. Ask the group members to share any personal encouragement, challenge, or inspiration they received as they watched.

CHOICES ACTIVITY (5 MINUTES)

Ask group members to think back on how they responded to the passage of Scripture they studied this week. Encourage them to take a few minutes to complete the Choices activity found on page 93 as a way of making sure they are not just "hearers" but "doers" of the Word.

WRAPPING UP AND MOVING FORWARD (5 MINUTES)

Conclude by asking the group members to write out their prayers to God on page 95, focusing on what they need to do to prevail in prayer. Refer them to the Pre-Session Bible Study found on pages 100–109, which describes the Bible study assignment for session 6. Remind them to read the passage and complete the studies before the next session. Close in prayer.

SESSION 6

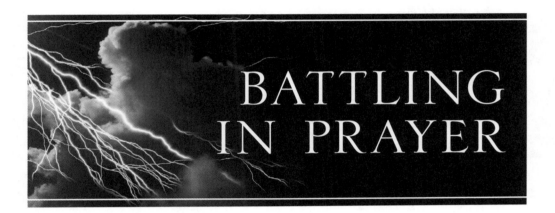

BATTLING IN PRAYER

For this final session, once again preview the video before your meeting and complete all the written exercises in the study guide. If possible, read the epilogue in *The Daniel Prayer* for more background information on the teaching covered during the session. Familiarize yourself with the session outline and gather the necessary materials. Remember also to pray for the group members who will be attending, asking God to help them view prayer as a battle in which they must take an active part.

SESSION OUTLINE (60 MINUTES)

I. Review of Pre-Session Bible Study (15 minutes)

   A. Study 1: Ephesians 6:10–11

   B. Study 2: Ephesians 6:12–13

   C. Study 3: Ephesians 6:14–15

   D. Study 4: Ephesians 6:16–17

   E. Study 5: Ephesians 6:18–20

II. Video Teaching (25 minutes)

    A. The battle is serious . . .

    B. Our armor is serious . . .

        1. Belt of truth

        2. Breastplate of righteousness

        3. Sandals of the gospel of peace

        4. Shield of faith

        5. Helmet of salvation

        6. Sword of the spirit

        7. Weapon of prayer

    C. The battle is subtle . . .

    D. The battle is spiritual . . .

III. Group Discussion (10 minutes)

    A. How does it change your view of prayer when you see it as a spiritual battle?

    B. What are some subtle things the enemy does to try to keep you from praying?

    C. How does the enemy try to convince you the battle is not serious?

    D. Why is it critical to wrap yourself in God's Word before confronting the enemy?

    E. In what ways does the Word of God serve as your weapon in the fight?

IV. Choices Activity and Wrapping Up (10 minutes)

REVIEW OF PRE-SESSION BIBLE STUDY (15 MINUTES)

Refer the group to their notes on pages 100–109. As time allows, have one member share the **facts** he or she drew from each verse (Step 2). Then have several different members share the following:

- The **lessons** they learned from each verse (Step 3).

- The most meaningful **question** they wrote out in response to Step 4, citing the verse on which the question was based.

- Their outstanding **takeaway** in Step 5.

Spend a few minutes of this time allowing the participants to reflect on what God has taught them during the study. What have they changed in their prayer habits? How have they started to pray their own Daniel Prayers for the people in their world?

VIDEO TEACHING (25 MINUTES)

Watch the teaching video for session 6. Refer the group members to the outline on page 110 and remind them there is space to take notes.

GROUP DISCUSSION (10 MINUTES)

Refer to the Group Discussion questions on page 111 to stimulate discussion on the topics presented during the video teaching. Ask the group members to share any personal encouragement, challenge, or inspiration they received as they watched.

CHOICES ACTIVITY AND WRAPPING UP (10 MINUTES)

Ask group members to think back on how they responded to the passage of Scripture they studied this week and then encourage them to take a few extra minutes to complete the Choices Activity found on pages 111–113 as a way of making sure they are not just "hearers" but "doers" of the Word. If time allows, encourage the group to share their responses. Conclude by asking group members to write out their prayers to God on page 114, focusing on what help they need from God as they battle in prayer. Encourage them to keep studying God's Word and spending time with the Lord each day in prayer. Then close in prayer yourself.

SIMPLIFIED AND ABBREVIATED BIBLE STUDY TRACK

For this alternate track, your group members will study only a few key verses together, and no weekly homework assignments will be required. At the start of each session, you will lead a short discussion of the facts, lessons, and most meaningful questions they discover from the verses they study. Make sure they pinpoint a takeaway from Step 5. You will then play the video (with the group members taking notes), and discuss the questions listed for this track. Your meeting time will need to be at least **45 minutes** in order to cover all the necessary material in this track.

SESSION 2
SIMPLIFIED STUDY

PREPARING FOR PRAYER

Preview the video for session 2 before your meeting. If possible, read the introduction and chapter 1 of *The Daniel Prayer* for more background information on the teaching covered during the session. Familiarize yourself with the session outline and pray for the participants, asking God to help them as they go through the steps on preparing for prayer.

SESSION OUTLINE (45 MINUTES)

I. Bible Study: Daniel 6:10 (10 minutes)

II. Video Teaching (18 minutes)

    A. A prepared place to pray . . .

    B. A prepared time to pray . . .

    C. A prepared atmosphere for prayer . . .

    D. A prepared attitude for prayer . . .

III. Group Discussion (12 minutes)

    A. What encouraged or challenged you in this study?

    B. What did you learn that was a new thought to you?

IV. Wrapping Up (5 minutes)

BIBLE STUDY (10 MINUTES)

Welcome any new participants, and then refer the group to the Bible study worksheet on pages 118–119. Ask one person to read the passage aloud and share the **facts** he or she can draw from it (Step 2). Then, as a group, discuss the following:

- The **lessons** they can learn from the verse (Step 3).

- The most meaningful **question** they can write out in response to Step 4.

- How they will **respond** to God's Word (Step 5).

VIDEO TEACHING (18 MINUTES)

Watch the teaching video for session 2. Refer the group members to the outline on page 120 and remind them there is space to take notes.

GROUP DISCUSSION (12 MINUTES)

Refer to the Group Discussion questions on page 120. Ask the group members to share any personal encouragement, challenge, or inspiration they received as they watched.

WRAPPING UP (5 MINUTES)

Conclude by asking the group members to consider writing out their prayers to God during the week, expressing their gratitude to the Lord in spite of the challenges or trials they are facing. Close your time together in prayer.

SESSION 3
SIMPLIFIED STUDY

PROMPTING
IN PRAYER

Preview the video for session 3 before your meeting. If possible, read chapters 2 and 3 of *The Daniel Prayer* for more background information on the teaching covered during the session. Familiarize yourself with the session outline and pray for the participants, asking God to help them as they go through the steps on being prompted to pray the Daniel Prayer.

SESSION OUTLINE (45 MINUTES)

  I. Bible Study: Daniel 9:2–3 (9 minutes)

 II. Video Teaching (22 minutes)

    A. Compelled by . . .
       1. Problems in the world
       2. Promises in God's Word

B. Centered on God . . .

   1. Privately

   2. Sincerely

   3. Desperately

   4. Humbly

III. Group Discussion (9 minutes)

   A. What encouraged or challenged you in this study?

   B. What did you learn that was a new thought to you?

IV. Wrapping Up (5 minutes)

BIBLE STUDY (9 MINUTES)

Welcome any new participants, and then refer the group to the Bible study worksheet on pages 124–125. Ask one person to read the passage aloud and share the **facts** he or she can draw from it (Step 2). Then, as a group, discuss the following:

- The **lessons** they can learn from the verse (Step 3).

- The most meaningful **question** they can write out in response to Step 4.

- How they will **respond** to God's Word (Step 5).

VIDEO TEACHING (22 MINUTES)

Watch the teaching video for session 3. Refer the group members to the outline on page 126 and remind them there is space to take notes.

GROUP DISCUSSION (9 MINUTES)

Refer to the Group Discussion questions on page 127. Ask the group members to share any personal encouragement, challenge, or inspiration they received as they watched.

WRAPPING UP (5 MINUTES)

Conclude by asking the group members to consider writing out their prayers to God during the week, focusing on the promises from the Bible that they need to pray back to the Lord. Close your time together in prayer.

SESSION 4
SIMPLIFIED STUDY

PLEADING IN PRAYER

Preview the video for session 4 before your meeting. If possible, read chapters 4–6 of *The Daniel Prayer* for more background information on the teaching covered during the session. Familiarize yourself with the session outline and pray for the participants, asking God to help them as they go through the steps on pleading in prayer.

SESSION OUTLINE (45 MINUTES)

  I. Bible Study: Daniel 9:4–5 (8 minutes)

 II. Video Teaching (25 minutes)

    A. Pleading with confidence based on your covenant relationship with God . . .

    B. Pleading with confidence based on God's character . . .

       1. God's faithfulness

       2. God's righteousness

       3. God's goodness

       4. God's greatness

    C. Pleading with contrition . . .

III. Group Discussion (9 minutes)

    A. What encouraged or challenged you in this study?

    B. What did you learn that was a new thought to you?

IV. Wrapping Up (3 minutes)

BIBLE STUDY (8 MINUTES)

Refer the group to the Bible study worksheet on pages 130–131. Ask one person to read the passage aloud and share the **facts** he or she can draw from it (Step 2). Then discuss the following:

- The **lessons** they can learn from the verse (Step 3).

- The most meaningful **question** they can write out in response to Step 4.

- How they will **respond** to God's Word (Step 5).

VIDEO TEACHING (25 MINUTES)

Watch the teaching video for session 4. Refer the group members to the outline on page 132 and remind them there is space to take notes.

GROUP DISCUSSION (9 MINUTES)

Refer to the Group Discussion questions on page 133. Also alert group members to the "List of Sins" mentioned by Anne during the teaching (pages 147–149 of their guides). Ask them to share any personal encouragement, challenge, or inspiration they received as they watched.

WRAPPING UP (3 MINUTES)

Conclude by asking the group members to consider writing out their prayers to God during the week, focusing on what they need to do to plead in prayer. Encourage them to read through the "List of Sins" three times, as suggested in the video. Close your time together in prayer.

SESSION 5
SIMPLIFIED STUDY

PREVAILING IN PRAYER

Preview the video for session 5 before your meeting. If possible, read chapters 7–9 of *The Daniel Prayer* for more background information on the teaching covered during the session. Familiarize yourself with the session outline and pray for the participants, asking God to help them as they go through the steps on prevailing in prayer.

SESSION OUTLINE (45 MINUTES)

I. Bible Study: Daniel 9:21–23 (10 minutes)

II. Video Teaching (18 minutes)

   A. God answers prayer immediately . . .

   B. God answers prayer ultimately . . .

   C. God answers prayer specifically . . .

III. Group Discussion (12 minutes)

   A. What encouraged or challenged you in this study?

   B. What did you learn that was a new thought to you?

IV. Wrapping Up (5 minutes)

BIBLE STUDY (10 MINUTES)

Refer the group to the Bible study worksheet on pages 136–137. Ask one person to read the passage aloud and share the **facts** he or she can draw from it (Step 2). Then discuss the following:

- The **lessons** they can learn from the verse (Step 3).

- The most meaningful **question** they can write out in response to Step 4.

- How they will **respond** to God's Word (Step 5).

VIDEO TEACHING (18 MINUTES)

Watch the teaching video for session 5. Refer the group members to the outline on page 138 and remind them there is space to take notes.

GROUP DISCUSSION (12 MINUTES)

Refer to the Group Discussion questions on page 138. Ask the group members to share any personal encouragement, challenge, or inspiration they received as they watched.

WRAPPING UP (5 MINUTES)

Conclude by asking the group members to consider writing out their prayers to God during the week, focusing on what help they need to do to prevail in prayer. Encourage the group members to keep studying God's Word and spending time with the Lord each day in prayer. Then close in prayer yourself.

SESSION 6
SIMPLIFIED STUDY

BATTLING IN PRAYER

Preview the video for session 6 before your meeting. If possible, read the epilogue of *The Daniel Prayer* for more background information on the teaching covered during the session. Familiarize yourself with the session outline and pray for the participants, asking God to help them as they go through the steps on battling in prayer.

SESSION OUTLINE (45 MINUTES)

I. Bible Study: Daniel 10:12–13 (8 minutes)

II. Video Teaching (25 minutes)

    A. The battle is serious . . .

    B. Our armor is serious . . .

        1. Belt of truth

        2. Breastplate of righteousness

        3. Sandals of the gospel of peace

        4. Shield of faith

        5. Helmet of salvation

        6. Sword of the spirit

        7. Weapon of prayer

    C. The battle is subtle . . .

    D. The battle is spiritual . . .

III. Group Discussion (9 minutes)

    A. What encouraged or challenged you in this study?

    B. What did you learn that was a new thought to you?

IV. Wrapping Up (3 minutes)

BIBLE STUDY (8 MINUTES)

Refer the group to the Bible study worksheet on pages 142–143. Ask one person to read the passage aloud and share the **facts** he or she can draw from it (Step 2). Then discuss the following:

- The **lessons** they can learn from the verse (Step 3).

- The most meaningful **question** they can write out in response to Step 4.

- How they will **respond** to God's Word (Step 5).

VIDEO TEACHING (25 MINUTES)

Watch the teaching video for session 6. Refer the group members to the outline on page 144 and remind them there is space to take notes.

GROUP DISCUSSION (9 MINUTES)

Refer to the Group Discussion questions on page 145. Ask the group members to share any personal encouragement, challenge, or inspiration they received as they watched.

WRAPPING UP (3 MINUTES)

Conclude by asking the group members to consider writing out their prayers to God during the week, focusing on what they need to do as they battle in prayer. Close your time together in prayer.

ABOUT THE AUTHOR

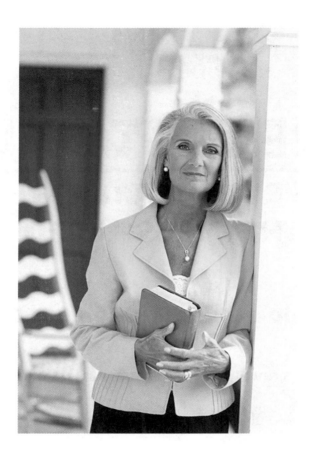

Called "the best preacher in the family" by her father, Billy Graham, Anne Graham Lotz is an international speaker and the bestselling and award-winning author of numerous books, including *Jesus Followers*, *Jesus in Me*, and *Just Give Me Jesus*. Anne is the president of AnGeL Ministries in Raleigh, North Carolina, and the former chairperson for the National Day of Prayer Task Force.

From the Publisher

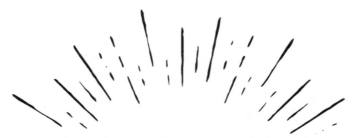

GREET STUDIES

ARE EVEN BETTER WHEN THEY'RE SHARED!

Help others find this study:

- Post a review at your favorite online bookseller.

- Post a picture on a social media account and share why you enjoyed it.

- Send a note to a friend who would also love it—or, better yet, go through it with them.

Thanks for helping others grow their faith!

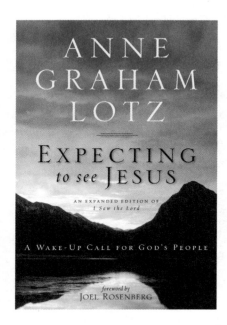

A WAKE-UP CALL FOR GOD'S PEOPLE

In this nine-session small group Bible study (DVD/ digital video sold separately), Anne Graham Lotz delivers a new message from the Mount of Olives in Israel and issues a wake-up call using the signs of Jesus' return.

EMBRACING THE GOD-FILLED LIFE

Follow author Anne Graham Lotz in this seven-session small group video Bible study (DVD/ digital video sold separately), on a journey through Abraham's life, and learn—as he did—how to live a life of joy and purpose in the midst of struggle and doubt.

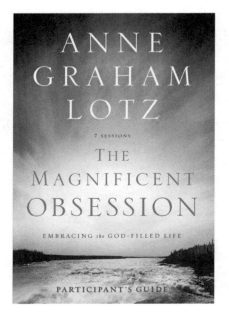

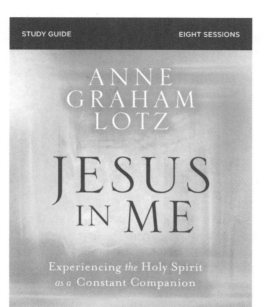

EXPERIENCING THE HOLY SPIRIT AS A CONSTANT COMPANION

Throughout this eight session video Bible study, you and your group will discover why the Holy Spirit is an essential part of the Christian life and how he speaks directly to you through the pages of your Bible.

REAL-LIFE LESSONS FOR IGNITING FAITH IN THE NEXT GENERATION

Join Anne Graham Lotz and Rachel-Ruth Lotz Wright for this five-session study focused on ways to ignite faith in the next generation, centered around your Witness, Worship, Walk, and Work. Intentionally following Jesus in these aspects of your daily life will make you more effective as you seek to pass the baton of faith.

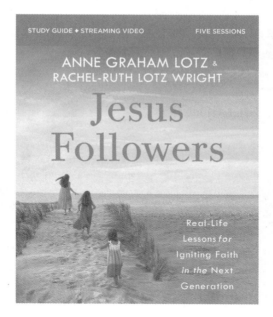